David Douglas Shannon

HELL *in the* HEAD

My War with a Brain Tumor and Other Evil Things

Hell in the Head
My War with a Brain Tumor and Other Evil Things
by David Douglas Shannon

KENILWORTH HOUSE PUBLISHING
LOS ANGELES USA
PO Box 1405
Los Angeles, CA 90078

Cover Photography: Michael Kurtz

Library of Congress Cataloging-in-Publication Data

Shannon, David Douglas
Hell in the head: my war with a brain tumor and other evil things
ISBN: 978-0-615-64201-7

Printed in the United States of America

To: The Crookedsmilers

ABOUT THE AUTHOR

David Shannon grew up in Pittsburgh, PA and graduated from Point Park University with a degree in Journalism. He spent the next 20 years as a marketing executive eventually leaving to establish a career in acting. He is now a freelance writer living in Los Angeles with his thoughts. This is his first published book.

AUTHOR'S NOTE

I have intentionally left the medical providers nameless in this account. While each did his or her job as they were expected (some better than others), perhaps they didn't go far enough and left too much unsaid. I am no one to judge, however, because I don't fully understand medical protocol. I'll leave that judgment up to you, the reader.

ACKNOWLEDGEMENTS

While there are a bunch of folks that I thanked at the conclusion of this story, there are two that I would like to thank up front. The first thanks goes to Barnetta Lange, who recently passed away, for sending me off in the right direction. The second thanks goes to the San Diego Writing Center, which no longer exists, for helping me take all the jumbled thoughts in my brain and put them on paper.

CONTENTS

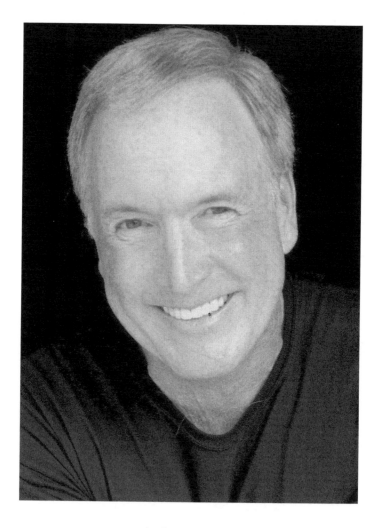

David Shannon, June 2006
Photography by Chance Miller

PREFACE

I was my smile. It was big, charming, and expensive. I suppose it had to do with my Irish roots and some fine dental work. I don't have it anymore. It's gone, and with it, the easy going charm. I lost it on December 3, 2007. I picked that date because it would have been my dad's 94th birthday. No other reason. It just seemed like a good time to take care of the thing. Of course, at the time, I didn't realize that my life as I knew it would come to an end that day.

Well-meaning people tell me that it could be worse. Yes, it could be worse. I read stories of cancer patients' pain and of men and women who have been wounded and disabled in combat and I realize just how much worse it could be. I function fairly well and if you were to pass me on the street, you would take me for just some other dope walking by. People in my life have all moved on and accepted my fate for me. But hell is a relative thing. It's not so much the tomorrow I believe in at night; it's the reality that greets me in the mirror the next morning. I'm reminded of it when retail clerks suddenly glance away uncomfortably. I'm reminded of it when people I meet spend an extra moment looking into my face to see the oddity. I'm reminded of it when I try to drink from a bottle and most of what I'm drinking spills out and onto my chin. I'm reminded of it when I look at "normal" pictures of me a few short years ago.

Hell in the Head

I asked my daughter to read some of this story. She said I didn't show any emotion. I didn't. I did have them though. A whole rollercoaster ride full. There were the funny times too – they made the ugly parts bearable. I've written about them. But slowly over the last three years, my soul was sucked dry. I didn't realize it at the time, but one day, I just didn't care anymore. Here's how it happened.

CHAPTER ONE

They Only Happen to Other People

December 3, 2007

A sudden wind snapped across the empty parking lot. A white paper bag, caught up in the gust, danced along the ground disappearing into the shadows. The early December morning was cold and dark and still. On a nearby street, a solitary bus roared by shattering the crystal silence. By Los Angeles standards, the air was fresh. I took in a deep calming breath. Somewhere deep within the recesses of thought, I heard the words "walk away." I brushed it off. My 25-year-old daughter, Britannia, stood patiently waiting by my side. She shuffled a little as if showing me the way I should be moving.

I glanced up at the building on the other side of the parking lot. It loomed upward into the lingering dark. St. Vincent's Hospital is a modern seven-story white stone and glass building. It sits just to the west of downtown Los Angeles in a seedy neighborhood of cheap motels, bullet-proofed liquor stores, and trash-littered streets. The hospital and the neighboring clinic stand as an architectural oasis in an otherwise gray and brown urban sprawl.

A thousand thoughts that should have been running through my mind, weren't. They had long before been pushed to a place where things didn't matter. Then, as if walking my last mile, my feet slowly began to shuffle toward the building. I was resigned to my fate. Of course it helped that I didn't know what my fate would be.

That walk started several months earlier in a nightclub in Long Beach. I was watching a Pink Floyd cover band. Toward the end of the night, there was a particularly high and intense guitar note during the song "Comfortably Numb", a song which in retrospect seems a bit ironic. Something suddenly seemed to be wrong. I had always been a little hard of hearing and had tinnitus, a ringing in one ear. But as I left the club that night things were different. My head was swirling in a hollow silence. I tried to pass it off as a temporary hearing loss due to the pounding my eardrums had just taken. But my worst fear had come to be as I woke the next morning. Most of my hearing was gone. I felt as though I was trying to hear with a tin wastebasket over my head. What made that harder to swallow was that it was my fault. I had failed to protect the hearing I had left.

Up until that point, I had been stumbling along through life fairly oblivious of my surroundings. After spending 20 years as a corporate marketing executive who was gradually losing his hearing and being unceremoniously nudged out because of it, I traded in my Mont Blanc for a Bic and pursued a career in acting. Well actually I pursued a career in writing; acting was supporting my writing habit

On my first day back to acting after the "incident," I quickly discovered that with my newly acquired hearing loss I was helpless on the chaotic and noisy sound stage of the TV show *House*. I couldn't understand simple directions, couldn't hear cues, and I was desperately trying to read lips. I struggled. Something as simple as walking down a hospital hallway on a dialogue cue became an impossible task.

Several months earlier, my doctor had given me a referral to an ENT (Ear, Nose, Throat doc) to determine if there was anything new that could help alleviate my tinnitus. Little did I know at the time that that would be the least of my worries. That night at home, after a long and frustrating day on *House*, I dug through piles of forgotten papers to rescue the referral. Within days I was in the office of the ENT. He prescribed tests – a hearing exam, a blood test, and an MRI.

The hearing test several days later in the audiologist's office showed that I had recently lost about 50% of my mid and high range hearing in what I call my "good ear." Hearing in my "bad ear" was a lost cause. I had only 11 % word recognition, meaning that I understood about one out of every 10 words which doesn't go too far in putting a meaningful sentence together. She told me that I was very hard of hearing. In that my vocabulary primarily consisted of "what," "huh," "pardon," and "again," I sort of suspected that I was a bit deaf. I just hadn't realized how deaf.

I have no idea what the blood test was for other than to annoy me.

I was also clueless about an MRI or the "Tube of Gloom" as I affectionately refer to it. I didn't research it and no one warned me. For those of you who are scheduled for an MRI and who are the least bit claustrophobic, ask your doctor for a Valium. Little did I know that tranquilizers are par for the course. And as another piece of advice, if a medical professional ever refers you to a procedure or a treatment that you are not familiar with, research it. Know what you are getting into. I didn't.

Hell in the Head

A very pleasant, smiling Indian radiologist greeted me to my doom and instructed me to lie on my back on a sliding table. He adjusted a vise and pads around my head so I couldn't move it and strapped me down so I couldn't escape – which I would have. He slid the table into the Tube of Gloom, a cold metal cylinder. It was peaceful for a moment. Then all hell broke loose. Drums pounded. Lights flashed. I kept my eyes closed tightly. I didn't know if there was something that I wasn't supposed to see for fear that it would melt my brain. After about 10 minutes of terror, I took a chance and peeked. Much to my relief, I realized that I wasn't risking brain damage. Above me at eyelevel was a mirror that was slanted at an angle. In the reflection, I was looking down to the open end of the tube and across the room to a window. Behind the window, the technician was working in a darkened room over a control panel. The lights of the monitors cast a sinister glow over his thin face. He looked intensely evil. I watched for awhile while he peered intently into the monitors. He seemed to be bothered. I didn't like that. I closed my eyes to hide from my thoughts.

Suddenly the lights and the pounding stopped and the table was sliding out. I was free, planning what I was going to have for lunch. No such luck. The technician tied my arm off with a rubber cord, raised a gleaming metal syringe filled with an evil potion, and injected it into my arm. I wondered how long it would take before everything went black. Then he did something really ugly. He slid me back into the cylinder for more mind-numbing claustrophobic torture. Soon the pounding and the flashing was again going full blast.

Eventually, the test that seemed to go on for ever, came to a merciful end. The table was sliding out and I would soon have my freedom.

But there was something wrong. The pleasant smiling Indian radiologist wasn't smiling anymore. Instead, he was solemn, serious. He said a very practiced, undertaker-type goodbye. I passed it off as he must have indigestion or something.

In his office the next day, the ENT's words hit me with a nasty sucker punch. He called it something else initially and showed me the white glob on my MRI film, the same white mass that the technician had seen. He calmly rambled on, describing the prognosis, the treatment and the options. I heard little. "Brain tumor" was screaming in my head. It was the last thing I had expected to hear that day. It was the last thing I had expected to hear in my life. Brain tumors happen to other people.

I sat in my car after leaving his office and stared out the window. Life moved along on that quiet Beverly Hills side street on the beautiful late summer day as if nothing had happened. But it had. I was suddenly different than other people passing by. I lost track of time. It really didn't matter. My peaceful life had just been rocked to its core, greater than I had realized at the time.

I had an Acoustic Neuroma – a wicked thing for something that sounded so pleasant. Now there are those who find great orgasmic pleasure in going into intricate technical detail describing an Acoustic Neuroma. I don't. Complicated medical terms are like algebra to me. It hurts my head to think about them. But in my simple guy kind of way, I'll try to describe an Acoustic Neuroma (sometimes called a vestibular schwannoma – beats me why they can't call it just one thing. Or more commonly called an AN). The brain is the command center with all these switches that control things that have wires running from them to various parts of the body. In this certain area near the inner ear, wires from the brain pass through – sort of like a fuse box. Those wires send brain signals to the inner ear for balance and hearing and to the face muscles to control movement – like a smile. The fuse box place is where the trouble started. A tumor (benign) took up residence there creating havoc with the signals running through the wiring – sort of short-circuiting things making for uneven balance, bad hearing and a messed up face. Now it wouldn't be so bad if that was all the mischief they caused, but the tumors grow and cause real trouble – like strokes and even death. These are not good things.

That may or may not be a good way of describing an AN, but that's as close as I'm going to get. My tumor had been growing there for the past 10 years – which I attributed every dumb thing I did during that time to it – and I made sure to let everyone know. Now here's the kicker. There are only about 3,000 Acoustic Neuromas diagnosed in the US each year. A cozy, exclusive club. But as a bit of a warning, that club may not be so cozy. Those are just the diagnosed tumors. A study indicates that autopsy results have shown that sub-clinical ANs (undiagnosed) are present in up to 1% of people. I believe what that is saying is that there are a lot of people who don't know they've got the thing. That's an Acoustic Neuroma in a nutshell – my little "hell in the head."

And so the dubious adventure began. I got a hearing aid and for the first time in my life, I realized that I actually had been quite deaf even as a child and never knew what other people heard. All those "you're not paying attention" were actually because I just didn't hear. Suddenly with my top-of-the-line discreet behind-the- ear model aid, I could finally hear the way I was supposed to (albeit a bit processed). The first thing I noticed when I put the hearing aid in was that the audiologist was screaming at me. I soon found that most people scream. The next thing I noticed was the office air-conditioning. How any one could concentrate on work with that thing rattling around was beyond me. But the biggest shock came when I stepped out the door and onto the street. The world is loud! My God, no wonder people go nuts with all that racket. I thought it was just a low rumble, not an explosion of noise. There were the pleasant discoveries though. While taking an exploratory adventure around the neighborhood later that day, I found that dry leaves crackle underfoot when you step on them. I also realized for the first time that the local CVS had a PA system that played music. I really didn't know that. But the biggest surprise was hearing a water fountain for the first time – the sound of a splash was a bit more crystal sounding than I had thought. Of course I soon discovered the greatest feature of the hearing aid – I could turn it off whenever I wanted to.

The ENT had referred me to a local ear clinic for consultation. The place was just a few miles down the street from where I lived and, as I later discovered, it was the top clinic in the world specializing in Acoustic Neuromas. Such convenience. I scheduled an appointment with the doctor who would usher me into the whimsical AN world. Two weeks later I met with him. He confirmed that I had the tumor and estimated it to be one and a half to two centimeters in size. Since I am sure I missed math class the day metrics was being taught, I guessed that to be anywhere between the size of a pea and a bowling ball.

He spelled out my options. I could wait to see how fast the tumor was growing or I could have surgery to have it removed. It was too big for radiation. The problem with waiting, as he explained, was that the tumor could press on the brainstem causing a stroke and potentially death. That death thing caught my attention. I quickly opted for surgery and agreed on a date.

The next two months were a jumble of medical terms, insurance, notifying, scheduling, preparing, and panicking. In retrospect, knowing what I know now, panicking would have topped that list. Instead I was blissfully naïve concerned more with what insurance would cover.

As I learned during the consultation at the clinic this thing was going to cost a lot. Real big bucks. More than the Aston Martin I dreamed of owning. The surgery was a big deal and more complex than I imagined. For some odd reason I just figured that if they wanted to get something from the inner ear, they'd just use the hole God had provided – the ear canal. Not so. As I learned in research, they put a hole in your head. At that point I stopped researching. I really didn't want to know anymore. As far as I was concerned, the thing would be magically removed.

In the process of the surgery, not only would the tumor be removed, but so would the balance nerve, the hearing nerve and the ever capricious facial nerve may be "slightly" affected. In other words, hearing would be gone in that ear (what was left of it), the balance nerve in the other ear would compensate (in theory), and there might be some facial weakness. That's sort of like saying an atomic bomb could cause some damage.

I'm often asked by others if I noticed any particular symptoms prior to being diagnosed with a brain booger. Actually, there wasn't much of anything. They say that the tinnitus – the ringing in the ear like coming out of a loud concert – is an indicator but not a definite correlation. I suppose the only real symptom had to do with my balance. My daughter pointed it out to me in retrospect. For my entire life, I had walked with long purposeful strides. But in the year leading up to the discovery of the tumor, she had noticed that I had been walking with shorter, tentative steps. And I noticed whenever I did sit-ups on an inclined bench, I would get dizzy when I finished and stood up.

Then there was the *Woman's Murder Club* incident. I played the first murder victim on the TV show. Only the episode never aired – something about a change in cast members. But I did get the picture of me below. Anyway, I spent an entire day lying dead on a wood floor of a mansion in a pool of blood which was actually red corn syrup that caused my face to stick to the floor. At the end of the day when the filming stopped, I stood up. Reeling from the dizziness caused by the yet unknown brain tumor, I staggered around the room like Frankenstein's monster and out a door where I stepped on a tarp covered swimming pool only to lurch and lunge even further to the delight of the production crew. I think even Angie Harmon had a bit of a chuckle. Regaining my composure, I staggered off into the night believing that it was just an old age thing unaware of the future that was looming ahead later that year.

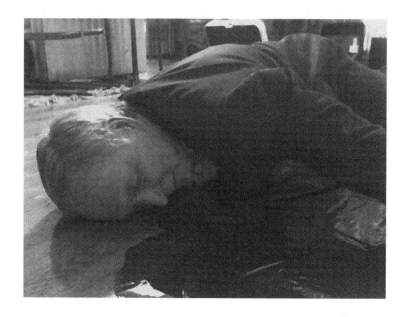

Dead Dave, "Women's Murder Club" March 2007

I spent the months leading up to surgery doing my best to prepare. I reasoned that if my balance was to be an issue, I would do all that I could to get in good balance condition. I kayaked, ran, bicycled, and hiked. I tackled the insurance monster. There were some folks who were helpful and some who were not so helpful, especially one who had a vested interest in my surgery. Beats me why some people just don't get that patient-provider customer service thing. I notified friends, family, and pretty much anyone who would listen and even those who didn't want to listen. This was important. At least it was to me.

There were a few memorable days leading up to the surgery. A week before the grand event, I went through pre-surgery counseling, a pre-surgery physical, signed releases and waivers, and turned in my pull-the-plug statement. It did ease my concerns a bit, especially about that hole in the head stuff.

The next day, Thanksgiving, my daughter and I ran the Turkey Trot 5K along the ocean in Long Beach. We would do it again two years later under different circumstances. We had dinner together in the evening. We took pictures. They would be the last taken of me smiling.

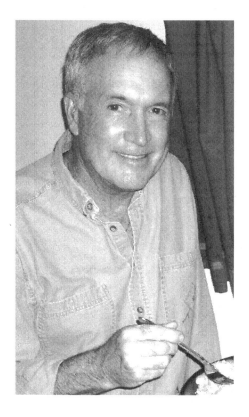

Thanksgiving 2007, the four glasses of wine last smile

On November 30, I said my goodbyes to the cast and crew of *Brothers and Sisters* and walked through the rain from the stage to the

Disney Studios "Zorro" parking lot expecting to be back in a couple of months when I had recovered and the Writer's Guild strike had ended. Little did I know at the time that I was exiting my acting career stage right.

I spent most of the day before my surgery alone. I went to church in the morning and spent time talking and praying with Jeff, the associate pastor. I left church to take a last hike up Runyon Canyon. The canyon, running from the streets of Hollywood to the top of the Hollywood Hills, features several steep trails that are favorites of fitness buffs, actors, and dog walkers. By city standards, it's a challenging climb. Less than an hour after I set out, I reached the top above Mulholland Drive and had worked off a lot of anxiety. Still, as I looked out over the peaceful view from the mountains to the city to the ocean, a feeling of dread crawled across me. I shook it off. When it finally came down to it, my biggest concerns were whether I would have to pay the hospital deductible and how I could go a whole month without blowing my nose – it would blow open the hole in my head.

That evening, I had my last meal of crab cakes with my daughter and my friend, Cindy at her California Pizza Kitchen in Tarzana. It would be two days before I could eat again. The meal was a great one to go out with. Unfortunately, that was the last of a pleasant evening. Noisy neighbors kept me up most of the night and by morning my nerves were rattled again. They would be a source of madness for the next year.

My date with the drill (or however it's done, still don't want to know) was scheduled for 7:00 AM. In order to be there in time for all the prep stuff, I had to be there at 5:00 before the hospital started cranking. Britannia and I spent quiet time alone in the Admissions Room doing crossword puzzles and reading magazines. Eventually I was taken back to a prep room where I traded my street clothes for a standard issue gown and leggings.

Cindy joined us. Cindy was a long time friend. She had been there through a lot of my big people life. And I trusted her with my life – literally – well actually my death. I had given her power-of-attorney to pull the plug in the event that I vegged during surgery. After all, she did put a cat down once.

One of the doctors was late so we waited there a bit talking. By that time I was getting antsy and ready to get on with things. Everything would be fine. Yep, just fine and dandy.

Finally my time had come and I was wheeled out of the prep room on the gurney and onto an elevator. As we exited the elevator, I was stunned by the flood of sunlight. Unlike the cavernous corridors leading to surgery rooms in other hospitals that I had the misfortune of visiting, St. Vincent's surgery wing was on the top floor surrounded by floor to ceiling windows. I said goodbye to Britannia and Cindy and as I was being wheeled down the hall I watched the morning sun streaming in over the Los Angeles skyline. It was a comforting moment at the end of a bumpy two-month journey.

I was taken to a pre-op room where everyone scurried around washing and scrubbing. I was given a bit of Valium which made the morning smiley. Then for some odd reason, one of the doctors asked me which side my tumor was on.

"Hey, you just gave me Valium. How do I know?"

I mustered up all the seriousness I could and told them the right side. I guessed right. He marked it with an "X." As I later found out, most pre-surgery physicals are done the day before surgery. The doctor marks the "X" then. Since my physical was a week before, they figured it would be gone by the time my surgery rolled around.

As surgeries go for a patient, it was typical. One minute I was carrying on a pleasant drug-induced conversation with the anesthesiologist and the next minute I was someplace else with bandages and tubes and wires and blinking and beeping things all over the place with an oxygen mask strapped over my face and a big bandage wrapped around my head. I made a wild guess that I was alive and out of surgery. I was. Over four hours of it. Within minutes Britannia and Cindy were by my side in the ICU as we carried on a pleasant "I'm alive" conversation and I managed to sing a little "Swing low, sweet chariot."

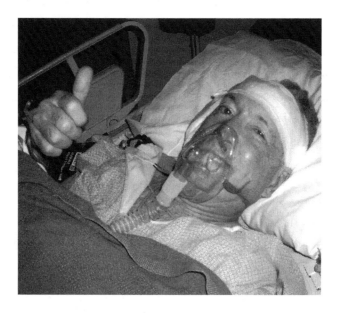

Just out of surgery in the ICU, December 3, 2007

The doctors stopped by. They assured me they got the tumor. They did mention, however, that the tumor had been sticky and that as it was removed, my facial nerve was stretched. It would cause temporary facial paralysis but I would be "fine" in a month or two. I gave it little thought. Three years later I give it a lot of thought.

Soon I was alone in the care of my ICU nurse. The first thing I noticed was that the hole in my head didn't hurt. The next thing I noticed was that everything else did. My neck was in agony. They must have had my head completely twisted around to get at the tumor during surgery. My eye was in pain. Due to the paralysis on the side of my face, I couldn't close my eye and it had become dry and painful. I also realized that I was itchy all over my neck and shoulders from a large red rash. It felt like a bad sunburn or poison ivy or both. I'm guessing that I had been allergic to the anti-bacterial shampoo I had been given to wash my hair and face with in the morning. And on top of that, I was dying of thirst. Some people have nausea post-AN surgery. Some have headaches. I had my own set of demons to deal with. I immediately launched into begging for ice chips. They allowed them sparingly for fear that too many would cause me to vomit.

"Hey lady, give me the damn ice chips. I promise not to vomit."

I begged for eye drops. I couldn't get enough. Finally, with all the issues, I gave up and decided to fix it with pain medication.

St. Vincent's Hospital has a pain chart that describes your level of pain on a one through 10 scale; 10 being the greatest pain. I figured the top pain medication would take care of everything so I requested the 10 stuff. Mistake. The 10 medication is Dilaudid. The street name for Dilaudid is "Drug Store Heroin." The first thing I noticed was that my body was slowly rising from the bed dangerously closing in on the ceiling. Then suddenly I was soaring around the ICU in a euphoric trip down futuristic lane hallucinating little gremlins. That might sound like fun. But it was more like too much fun. After a couple of hours bouncing off the ceiling and walls like a aimless helium balloon, I landed and swore off the 10, settling on the five stuff and went back to itching, aching and thristing all while worrying about my catheter removal. That was day one.

I had a restless first night being prodded, monitored, poked, and tested while sucking on blessed ice chips. My eye had become the biggest issue and as I discovered, would be an issue for months to come and occasionally to this day. They gave me a moisture chamber patch to put over my eye. It kept the eye drop goop they were putting in my eye from drying out so quickly.

I spent the next day in a catatonic haze – the post anesthetic effects – napping in between being tested and poked. Then the dreaded moment came. The catheter removal. I had briefly considered the 10 stuff in advance but wasn't up to another wild ride.

I looked the nurse in the eyes and asked, "Will this hurt?"

She said a very practiced, "No."

She lied.

Finally, in the evening I was mercifully taken to my hospital room. I settled into a few days of reading, daytime TV, pizza commercials, hospital food, and being startled every few minutes to have my vitals checked. I'm sure a simple occasional "Are you OK?" would have worked just fine. I had visits from actor buddies, James and Freddy. Britannia and Cindy stopped in regularly. My biggest issue was my eye

– by then a dry, painful, gel-gooped, moisture chamber-covered mess. And I was tired. Real tired.

The third day, with a physical therapist's help, I began walking around the halls. Now with only one balance nerve left, the walks could be compared to walking the deck of a rolling ship not quite certain where and when foot and deck would meet. Britannia would regularly take me for hall walks. Everyone, including me, was amazed at how well I was walking – a little wobbly – but handling it. That was in the less-than-sensory-stimulating confines of the hospital. As I was to later discover, outside, in the frantic city world, that stroll on the deck was more like a wildly drunken lurching and lunging on a ship in the middle of a hurricane.

Friday finally rolled around and I was ready to be freed from captivity to eat food with taste. Later that night, while wolfing down a plate of nachos, I found out that it wasn't the hospital food that lacked taste. I had lost mine. Something that everyone had failed to mention as a side-effect. It would be months before I began to barely taste. But eating wasn't what it was cracked up to be. Because of my facial paralysis, I ended up chewing on my cheek and tongue more than I did the food.

As Britannia wheeled me out of the hospital into the gray, drizzly morning, she commented that with my toboggan cap, patch over my eye, and my crooked palsy smile that I looked like a pirate. It would be a common theme among AN patients as I was to learn.

For a fleeting moment it felt good to be out in the fresh air. But that feeling quickly faded. As I sat hunched over in my wheelchair at curbside in the rain waiting for Britannia to get her car, I looked out at the parking lot. Just days earlier, the morning had been cold and crisp when I had arrived. Everything was clear. Now in the swirling gray mist, I saw only shadows drifting silently through a veil of obscurity. I looked hard across the parking lot for Britannia's car anxious to get out of the rain and to go home. In the cold, damp air, a shiver ran up my back and I suddenly felt very alone. As a rain drop fell from my cap and splashed across my cheek, an odd thought ran across my mind – something wasn't right.

CHAPTER TWO

A Cold Slap of Reality

January 28, 2008

The rides had dried up. I really couldn't expect everyone to be my perpetual chauffeur. I had thought I would be driving by then but it had been two months since my surgery and my brain was still a mess. Fortunately the clinic and I were on the same bus line – there would be no need to make a connection that would add to my already creeping confusion. I had yet to undertake the public transportation adventure, but things weren't getting any better, I needed answers, three miles was too far to stagger, so I had to chance the Los Angeles Metro system.

I hate to look like a rookie. It's so uncool and unbecoming. Just like meeting the Queen, I was sure there was some protocol for riding the bus. I did a little online research. What I discovered was the one-way fare would be $1.25. Nothing else. I guessed I would have to figure the rest of it out on the fly.

So with a dollar and a quarter tightly clutched in one hand and a cane in the other, I ventured out into the cold, gloomy morning to walk the block from my place to the bus stop. I had driven by the stop many times before seeing the desperate souls standing there as if they knew that this was all life had to offer. Now I would become one of them. I would join their bus stop huddle and blend in. Well, not quite. I live in a very ethnically diverse neighborhood of Koreans, Hispanics, blacks and a smattering of white actors and bums. The actors drive and the bums stick to the alleys. Tallish white guys with canes don't blend in. And I didn't. Suspicions arose. I felt like an undercover immigration guy.

So there I stood at the bus stop in front of the two-level strip center with the original New York pizza place from Seoul, the token cell phone store, the two karaoke bars, the karaoke coffee shop, and a couple of places I had no idea what the were because their signs were in Korean, with my new compatriots as we waited on the number 16 bus that ran from Beverly Hills to downtown LA and back.

No one spoke except the bleary-eyed, stubble-bearded bums who stumbled out of the alley and slurred and drooled "change" with motley glove-covered out-stretched hands. I took my cue from the crowd and stared straight and clutched my dollar and quarter even tighter. Like spurned vampires, the bums retreated into the darkness of the nearby alley.

Then I began following the crowd. I glanced at my watch without noticing the time. Then I'd peer down Third Street into the imaginary distance. As the crowd did, so did I frequently repeat this. As I would later discover in my public transportation experiences in the years ahead, this ritual is believed to make the bus arrive sooner. I don't know if this truly worked. I think people were afraid that if they didn't do it, the bus wouldn't come. This time, at least, it worked.

Out of the mist three blocks away, Old 16, a big orange monster, crested a rise in the hill and roared into view. I tensed with rookie anticipation. Suddenly the crowd began to move in unison anticipating the bus's actual stopping place. Within seconds, the big machine rumbled to a stop. Several had misjudged and scurried back toward the door while those who had guessed right stood smugly in place. The doors hissed open.

Now I had thought the rules of chivalry would apply and that women would be allowed to board first, especially if they were pregnant or with small children (which most of them were). Not so. It was everyone for him or herself. As I eventually discovered, only the very old got a pass. I would soon find out why. I very gentlemanly, perhaps foolishly, was the last to board. Suddenly I was facing an impatient driver and a complex fare machine. In the long ago past, whenever I would ride a bus, I would drop my money in the fare box, the driver would give it a look over, then open a door at the bottom, and the money would disappear. Now with precious seconds ticking away that would reveal me as a rookie, I was now face-to-face an ATM-like device with small pads of paper attached all over the thing. Sensing my confusion the driver reached over and pointed to a slot.

"Dollar."

Then he pointed to a smaller slot.

"Quarter."

I looked at the dollar hoping that it was free of kinks and would go smoothly into the slot. I shoved it in. It spit it back out. I shoved it back in. It spit it back out. The driver glared at me. I glanced up. We were still at the stop because the light was red at the intersection. I had seconds. I pulled the dollar tight and slid it in again. This time it took. I quickly dropped the quarter into the slot and grabbed my cane to make the walk down the aisle. No sooner had I turned to walk than the light turned green and the bus lurched forward – so did I. With no meaningful balance, I was suddenly stumbling forward latching onto anything that I could find to steady me. Just before I fell, I grabbed onto the overhead rail. I might as well have screamed, "I'm a rookie."

As I lunged around past the front seats, I saw why the very old got a pass. The front seats were reserved for them. No one else was going to be able to sit there anyway. But beyond that, every seat was taken to the very back with just one place open in the middle of the back bench seat. I started making my way for it. Just then, the bus stopped and I went stumbling backward wildly swinging my cane around behind me to plant it any place solid. Several passengers looked at me wide-eyed in fear that I would land in their laps. I regained what little composure I had left and fell the remaining length of the aisle and into the seat. My neighbors on either side subtly scooted their butts away from me. I settled in just thankful that I was only going a short way.

It was a solemn event as we bounced along the three miles of rutted city streets passing an endless stream of brown, gray and dirty two-story storefront buildings. All the stores were the same nameless clothing and grocery stores, beauty parlors, taco places and check-cashers. Trash bins overflowed in rivers onto the sidewalks. Gang tags were painted on every available wall.

No one spoke. I don't know if they had nothing to say or no one spoke the same language or if they just wanted to imagine they weren't there. No one made eye contact. People by the window stared out the window. People sitting on the aisles stared at the floor. It was a moving mind morgue.

I watched carefully to learn the proper way of pulling the cord to signal a stop. I watched the proper way to exit the bus. The only thing to be heard was the rumble of the bus and the ping of the stop signal. We'd stop. A wool-covered gray and brown hovel would exit only to be replaced by an identical hovel getting on.

Then I saw it. Just as we began to climb a hill, St. Vincent's hospital loomed into view. Soon I could see the clinic across the street – the place where I would finally get my answers. I reached across my neighbors and pulled the signal cord. I didn't realize it, but there was a bus stop two blocks short of my intended stop. The bus came to a sudden stop. Since I pulled the stop cord, I felt obligated to get off. I carefully made my way to the door and down the steps to step out on the curb to discover something else that I had to deal with. One without much balance does not get off a moving bus and expect the ground to be still. I took one step and nearly fell over. Until my brain could catch up with its surroundings, I stood frozen in place, grinning sheepishly at passing cars, trying to look natural while doing it.

Eventually my brain and the sidewalk got into synch and I walked the two blocks up the hill to the clinic and my internist's office. It had been two months since my surgery, things weren't getting any better, and I wanted to know why. I got my answer.

"It could take a year, you know," he said as he looked at the floor avoiding my eyes.

There was a sudden awkward silence. Well, gee, I didn't know. I was told it would take one or two months. No one mentioned "year" in any conversation. Everything was unraveling in my head. The palsy, the lack of balance, the disorientation, the loneliness mess could take a year? Everything I had planned – the return to work, a financial recovery, living like I did before surgery, walking a straight line, smiling – just came crashing down in a big heap. I don't remember leaving his office, but I do remember the bus ride home was much grayer that day.

Recovery had been ugly from the first day back from the hospital. The noise from the neighbors was relentless. One of them had decided to take up the bass guitar. He learned two notes. He played them all night and only stopped to sleep during the day. I complained. He turned up the volume. I complained again. He played one note. The apartment management was useless.

There was a refrigerator repair scam. During my stay in the hospital, my refrigerator had opted not to work. All the food that I had meticulously stocked pre-surgery for the post-surgery recovery went bad. Someone arranged for a repair service to be there on my first day home. The guy took a quick look and said it was a burned out fuse box. Knowing less about refrigerators than I know about brain surgery and still under the influence of brain surgery, I decided to have it replaced for $150. Then with the help of Britannia and others, I restocked it… only to realize the fuse box repair didn't work, the refrigerator was once again not working, and the food once again went bad. With a great deal of effort, I encouraged the appliance repair company to return only to be told that it wasn't the fuse box that was the problem, it was the compressor – which would cost more than the refrigerator did. I asked for my fuse box money back. The guy at the appliance repair company said my check would be returned to me. He lied. After repeated attempts to get my money refunded, phone calls where I was hung up on in mid-sentence, I slowly wore out and gave up. I had to buy a new refrigerator from a bank account that was hemorrhaging with medical bills. A piece of advice – be careful with companies that are named "AAA-something." They know they're going to get their share of the business by being first and it doesn't matter what their reputation is – which by the way, according to various internet review sites, this one was horrendous.

Then there was the bad pizza experience. Throughout my stay in the hospital, I had been bombarded by TV commercials for a certain delivery pizza company. By the time I was released from the hospital, I craved pizza. So on the second night home, I ordered my favorite food online. I was finally going to be able to taste something. I waited. I waited some more. Finally I called the store. They told me it was on the way. I waited. I called back. They hung up on me. It took two hours to get that far. By now I was on a pizza mission. I was going to have pizza for dinner. I called another store and explained the situation. They assured me they would have a pizza to me within an hour. And they did. In just under an hour (three hours after I started the process) they delivered a cold, dried-out pizza that looked like it had been sitting out on a shelf for a day. I took a slice of it and sent it with a letter to the president of the company. He never responded. Thanks, John.

Dear Noisyneighboruselessapartmentmanagementripoffappliancecompanylamepizzadelivery, you just might want to think twice the next time you pull this kind of #@$%. It might just end up in print.

Signed, Nowweareeven

This was something I really didn't need.

And I was incredibly tired. Nap time came frequently. I was so tired that I fell asleep on the kitchen floor while trying to make a sandwich. It just seemed like a reasonable place to take a nap.

There was the good. Acting friends from the TV show *Alias*, Freddy and Justin, took me for the initial follow-up doctor's visits. Justin treated me to a burger. As I quickly discovered, with a half-paralyzed face, I couldn't get my mouth open wide enough to take a bite out of it without some of it falling back out of my mouth. Not a pleasant experience. To this day, I still have problems, which is the reason why I don't eat in expensive restaurants where I would gross-out high-paying customers as well as watching half of my costly dinner end up on the floor. I also discovered something else that day as we left the burger place. Sitting lower on the horizon to get a good clean shot, the winter sun pierced my bad eye with a razor laser. I couldn't close my eye. I couldn't even squint to protect it from the blinding sun. All I could do was scream and wave my cane at the sun. If I hadn't been on the streets of LA, I am sure I would have looked quite odd. I, instead, looked quite natural.

Looking back on this moment, I remember how bad that really was. I suppose over time, I've pushed the really ugly stuff out of my head. In the early days post-surgery, it was the eye pain that I had suffered the most. The pain was relentless, my single focus for the first four months. It felt like sandpaper being scraped back and forth over my eyeball. Because of the facial paralysis, my eye wouldn't completely close. During the day, I would frequently have to close my eye with my finger. At night, when I would be sleeping, my eye would still be partially opened. To sleep somewhat peacefully, I would have to gob up my eye with some goop called Refresh Celluvisc lubricant eye drops and cover it with the moisture chamber. The moisture chamber was a clear plastic goggle surrounded by foam on the sides and held in place by an elastic band around my head. In theory, it prevented outside air from getting to my eye preventing it from becoming painfully dried out. In reality, it usually found its way to being tangled around my face during the night and end up covering my nose – which of course didn't need to be covered.

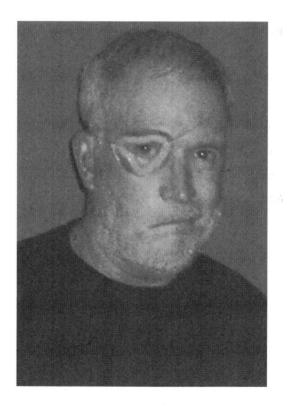

The dreaded moisture chamber, Christmas 2007

Another one of those nasty little eye things was the permanent contact lens that the ophthalmologist had given me to wear to protect my cornea from drying out. I had never worn contacts. That was a wise decision. The thing was scratchy and miserable. And like the moisture chamber, it generally found its way to somewhere it wasn't supposed to be – like my ear.

There were other eye issues. Because of the paralysis, my lower eyelid drooped looking as though my eye might fall from its socket. When I look back on those days, I'm actually amazed that I ventured out in public. I looked like a deranged Igor or Bloom County's Billthecat. Ack. My eye doctor suggested that I place a thin strip of tape under my lower eyelid and stretch it up into the corner to pull my eye back into a more reasonable place – although I don't know what looked more bizarre – a cartoon character or a self-made facelift. To this day, I still have some issues with my eye. In arid weather, it dries out and I have to use drops to moisturize it. But I am fortunate. There are other AN patients with far worse cases who have had to have gold weights and springs placed in their eyelids to help them close. It's not a pretty deal.

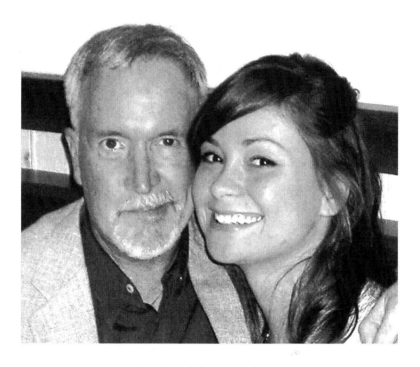

The "eye" with daughter, Britannia, Easter 2008

I had other guests in those early days. My acting casting agent, Jessica, stopped by for a visit bringing with her homemade Greek soup (it was the first thing and the last thing I tasted for some time). She also brought a bamboo plant, a gift from a casting director. Today it is twice the size it was three years ago. It measures my recovery. Slow but steady.

Two weeks after I returned home from the hospital, James (my acting buddy who had visited me in the hospital) stopped by and took me for a two-mile walk around my tree-shaded Hancock Park neighborhood. Hancock Park takes up about a four square mile area west of downtown

LA. It's filled with stately old mansions that occupy entire zip codes – the guest houses being larger than most ordinary houses. The sidewalks are wide and generally deserted, the perfect place to walk with an unsure step. I needed my cane but it was truly a major accomplishment. Today, I still walk those streets remembering the early days.

I spent my December days sleeping a lot and during waking moments getting ready for Christmas, sending out cards, and taking care of my eye. Britannia came to my place for Christmas. We had a great evening finishing it off with our traditional Roast Beef and Yorkshire pudding dinner. There was one particular irony during the day. Britannia took me to see the newly released *The Bucket List*. The irony being that I had worked on the movie as Jack Nicholson's stand-in earlier that year never realizing what a drastic turn my life would take by the end of the year. I still knew all the lines. Rob Reiner expected it of us. I even had a bit part as Jack's limo driver. It was like witnessing my old life for the first time post-surgery. But things were good and I was ready to be back to normal any day.

Then the rains started. I was trapped inside my LA apartment with the brick walls and wood floors. I was lonely. My balance had oddly gone from bad to worse. The Writer's Strike was ending and I had a face that couldn't go back to work and a balance system that was severely off-kilter – bad enough that I couldn't drive. I walked a lot. More rain.

Then came the financial issues. I was burning through my savings while living off a meager State Disability income. The State made a mistake and discontinued payments. Suddenly, with all the bills I had and medical expenses, I couldn't afford to buy food. No one realized that I was living on beans and a prayer. Then Dani, a lady I had befriended on the way to a Catalina Island movie shoot, must have caught on – maybe it was my pale cadaver look that tipped her off. For the three weeks I was waiting for the disability payments to resume, Dani would show up at my place every weekend with boxes of food. She was a life-saving angel. James also caught on and would casually bring great steaks that he had bought at the Naval commissary. I was getting along, still waiting for my recovery to end and to get back to work.

Then something odd happened a month after my surgery. During a visit to the ophthalmologist who had been caring for my eye, he asked me what at the time seemed like an innocuous question. He asked me if I had seen my doctor lately, the guy who did the surgery. I thought nothing of it at the time. I now realize that doctors don't casually ask you if you've seen your doctor. What he was saying was, "You need to see your doctor. There is something drastically wrong. Your whole world is a mess. And he's the one who is going to have to break the bad news!"

Two weeks later at the internists, I got the bad news. It could take a year to be back to normal. That changed things and made all the bad that was going on in my life even worse. I had planned to survive on State Disability for the two months. I needed to get back to work to make a living that I could reasonably live on. But an actor with only half a face that worked, with little balance, and couldn't even drive, was not going to make a living at acting. This wasn't the deal that I had bargained for and I was getting real tired living in my head. Little did I realize that the worst was yet to come.

CHAPTER THREE

Quasimoto Face

May 2, 2008

By now I had become accustomed to the look. The look with the practiced feigned smile that says, "I have some bad news for you. You're not going to like it, but if I keep smiling you'll think everything is OK." And the bad news was bad. My doctor informed me that it would take about two years before my face was about normal. What exactly was "about normal?" Something like Quasimoto? By this time I was really over bad news. First it was two months. Then it was a year. Now it's two years and only then would I be about normal. I had developed something called Synkinesis – a term I had heard about only two months earlier.

After my January visit to my internist where I first heard it could take a year to recover, I launched into an internet search looking for a better answer. The rains had come back, it was cold, and I was isolated and lonely. A gray depression was setting in. It was taking over my life and I knew if I didn't do something about it, it would be my life.

Then one morning in early February, I was poking around the internet when I stumbled across a site for the Acoustic Neuroma Association.

I clicked on one of the links called "support groups." Suddenly with the click of the mouse, I was whisked away to a discussion forum with ANers like me – fellow staggering, slack-faced, eye-patched pirates. Some even referred to themselves as pirates and named their imaginary ship "The Princess Batty Wench" (an apt name for post-AN surgery patients). It even had a captain and crew members with assignments.

Within minutes I was on-board communicating for the first time with other ANer's. It was a liberating experience to find that I was not alone with my struggles. I quickly became a member of the family, asking questions, giving advice, sharing experiences and learning. I had a lot of questions and they had a lot of answers. More answers than I had been getting to that point.

The crew of the PBW saw me through my cold winter loneliness. I found them to be witty, caring, and close-knit. I made many friends that I still have today. Since I had been nearly deaf most of my life, I discovered I could answer questions and give advice on hearing loss and tinnitus and hearing aids. I helped new members as they came aboard the Forum. And I learned that most folks on the Forum had post-surgery issues they were dealing with – many the same as mine. Balance was a common theme. They had even given it a term since the medical field lacked one (a condition the medical field doesn't seem to want to acknowledge). They called it Wonkyhead, a thing that can only be described as having a fishbowl for a head with water sloshing around inside. Some had it worse and relied on canes. There were those with eye problems like mine and several had had tiny weights placed in their eyelids to help them close. Fewer members had facial palsy issues; some of them severe and permanent, a few even had surgery to attempt to correct it. We shared experiences. For the first time I found that palsy could last years. I also heard about the twitches – tiny movement in the paralyzed face that signaled that nerves were reawakening.

Not long after that, in early March, it happened. James had been getting me out of the house whenever he could to take me hiking. We climbed local LA mountains. In early February, we had climbed the Verdugo Mountains. I needed a cane but it gave me a sense of accomplishment like I was moving upward and onward and not dwelling in a rut.

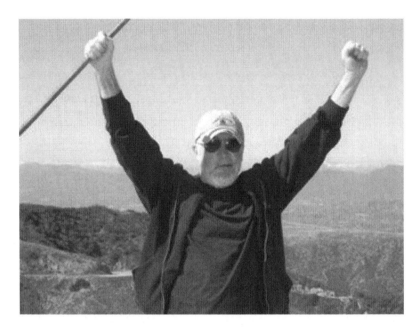

At the top of the Verdugo Mountains 2/7/08

This day in March, a month later, we hiked Rocky Peak high above the Simi Valley. Rocky Peak was a tough climb up a dusty, craggy, boulder-strewn trail. It was hot. It took us several hours. But we made it.

Later that evening, I was standing at my kitchen sink pouring a glass of wine in celebration of the hike and I felt it -- hardly noticeable at first -- little tingles near the corner of my mouth. They stopped. I anxiously waited. They started again. My nerves were coming back to life. My face and I were on the comeback trail.

March was a good month. I started getting small movement in my face. My eye was improving a little. Balance was still an issue, but the rains had stopped and I was getting out more often for long walks around the neighborhood. I discovered cheaper (and less crowded) public transportation shuttles that I used to get around more effectively.

Not long after I started getting the nerve twitches in my cheek, on March 15th I ventured out into an event in society. Obviously I had been out in public but not in a large gathering of humans. I was nervous and apprehensive and subtly looking for a way to get out of it. In the past, under normal circumstance, it would have been fun. But now I wasn't sure if I could handle the crowds and the disorientation and the sound.

For Christmas, Cindy had given me tickets to see the Moody Blues at the Nokia Theater in downtown LA. I had been a fan of the Moody Blues since they first hit the airwaves in the 60's. Their music was a rare combination of lush melody, energy and British Blues with a classical backdrop. Over the years, I had gone to their concerts whenever they were in town, even meeting them backstage after a show in Phoenix with, then, 10-year-old Britannia.

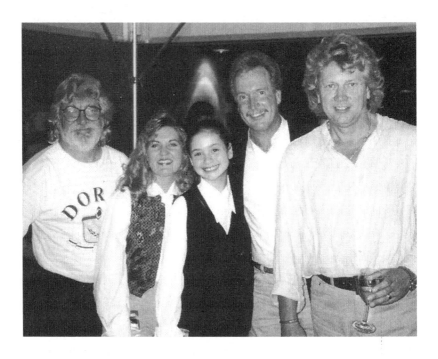

The Moody Shannons, Phoenix, September 24, 1994

So dressed in jeans and a black leather jacket (I tried to look the part), Cindy picked me up and we made the short trip downtown. As we entered the Nokia Theater complex, my balance and disorientation threw a fit as they suddenly had to deal with a large overwhelming building and the continuous flow of the crowd. They were going to have none of the proceedings. Sensing that I was having problems after I let out with an audible "Whoa," Cindy jumped in, took me by the arm and steered me through the maze of people and past the things that had been placed in front of me just to mess me up. We grabbed a beer and hotdogs before the show. It was the first time I had eaten in front of so many people and I did the best to conceal the food falling from my mouth – not very successfully. I'm sure I looked quite dapper.

This was the first Moody Blues concert I had been to in about 15 years. I was amazed to see how old their fans had become. They were balding and matronly, dressed in Polo sweaters and Dockers. In the early days, they would have been dressed in the finest silks and leather and suede with chains of gold and silver with stylishly coifed hair – the women dressed up too. And they all came in altered states – a condition that the Moody Blues music catered to. Now the only things altering our states were Viagra, Menopause, and out-of-whack hearing aids.

In a flurry of activity, the band took the stage – well they sort of hobbled on stage. They were no longer the brash rockers of yore. They played songs that we all knew, apparently better than they did since they forgot many of the words. I tried to figure out which worked better – leaving my hearing aid on with the processed sound or off to listen to natural sound. I don't remember what I settled on but I am quite sure a lot of the audience was dealing with the same dilemma. In spite of it all, the music was fun and nostalgic.

The band finished with their standard encore rocker, "Ride My Seesaw." They got a standing ovation – a bit slower and achy from all the arthritic knees. It was a gathering of past glory – a time when things were new and alive filled with promise and energy. Both band and fans were reliving a moment that would never be captured again. I wrote in the journal that I had been keeping since my surgery that on that day I said goodbye to my youth. I tend to be dramatic. Only this time I wasn't.

In late March, I discovered a new found freedom. I learned how to navigate the LA light rail train system and on a Saturday morning, I rode it to Britannia's place in Long Beach. We went to a local track and for the first time since surgery, with my daughter by my side to guide me, I ran. It wasn't anything special, more of a shuffle, but things were getting better. We did well enough that we decided to tackle our traditional Revlon "Run for the Cure" 5K in early May.

Of course not all the training leading up to the race went quite as planned. On April 20th, just a few weeks before the race, things went a little off. I made my normal morning trip to Britannia's on the subway to the train to the Long Beach shuttle across town to Britannia's place. We had a choice of two tracks to run on. One was Wilson High, a local Long Beach high school. The other was Los Alamitos high school. The good thing about the Los Alamitos track was that it was always open. The downside – it was a good ten miles away through heavy traffic. Wilson, on the other hand, was an easy mile away. But Wilson had a downside. The football-track-baseball complex was surrounded by a 100 foot fence topped with barbed wire. Now a 100 feet may be a slight exaggeration, but it might as well have been. (Actually, how high is 100 feet?). Wilson was also under lock and key unless a school sponsored event was taking place. During the fall and spring we could usually get into the track because the Wilson High baseball team would be playing a game on the adjoining ball field.

This particular day they weren't. But we lucked out. A Wilson High baseball player was taking batting practice, the gate was open, and we wouldn't have to make the long drive to the other track. While I don't remember what the routine was that day, we generally ran some interval training followed by a longer run. And as always, we wore iPods for inspirational running music. We finished the end of the long run, took off our ear buds and started walking a cool down lap. But something was different. It was quiet. There was no sound of a ball pinging off the end of a metal bat. He was gone. The batter was gone. We quickly gathered our stuff together and headed to the gate. It was locked. The #@&#%& had locked us in. Would it have been too hard for him to let us know that he was leaving? He had to know we were there. Apparently he must have had runner envy or something.

In any case, we were trapped behind a prison fence on one side and a school building on the other. Our cell phones were in the car. No one was around. No need to panic. No need to panic. Panic! We were doomed. We were going to starve to death. When the custodian showed up on Monday morning, he was going to find our decimated carcasses chowing down on the last of the Ding Dongs from the vending machine that we had broken into.

We reasoned (wrongly) that the only way out was through the school building since the sky-high prison fence wasn't an option. So we started our escape quest first through a locker room which we guessed was the boys since it had urinals. Then into a gym and up stairs that led to down stairs and into another locker room that we guessed was the girls since it didn't have urinals. No one could top us in smarts. Then we started down classroom hallways only to find the entryways chained closed. We discovered the lunch room with the precious vending machines that held our Ding Dongs was locked. I think we may have screamed. We spent the next hour frantically searching knowing full well that vultures were circling overhead.

Then, after nearly an hour of a panicked search, we found it. Just outside the cafeteria were trash dumpsters and discarded desks and a shorter fence of maybe 12 feet. I asked Britannia if she had ever climbed a fence. She said, no. At first I was shocked. But then I reckoned the only reason why anyone would climb a fence was to get into trouble – or get out of it. If you weren't facing either prospect, the opportunity probably would never have presented itself.

With my balance issue and her inexperience we would never have been able to scale the fence up one side and down the other. So we got creative. With the discarded desks, we built a step up to the dumpster. From there, we stacked more desks on top of the dumpster to the top of the fence where we could just roll over the top – in theory. One does not do too much thinking when one is trapped.

For some reason I thought Britannia should go first. I'm not sure what prompted that thinking or lack thereof. In retrospect, it would seem like the one who knew how to climb a fence should have gone first demonstrating to the other how it's done. Instead we chose to do it the dumb way. Britannia climbed her way through the desk and dumpster maze just reaching a little below the top to the point where she was close enough that she could pull herself up to straddle the top of the fence face down, arms and legs dangling on either side. Then after a little flailing around she announced in a mixture of chagrin, disgust and panic, "I'm stuck." I quickly tried scrambling up the first desk to her rescue only to lose my balance and fall backward on my butt. This of course was a dumb thing to do since I really had no plan once I reached her. The only thing left to do would be to talk her down. So for the next 10 minutes, I described in accurate detail the fine art of fence climbing – one step, one handhold at a time. Finally she made it as she dropped a few feet to the ground on the other side.

Now, with very little balance, it was my turn. I had climbed plenty of fences in my youth, both getting into and out of trouble. But then I had my full faculties, particularly balance. This would be a challenge. I don't remember much about the event except for grabbing at anything solid and secure. I misjudged the drop on the other side of the fence and landed hard but free of captivity. As we waved goodbye to the vultures, we had a good laugh – albeit a bit nervous. Looking at our rigged escape pile of desks on the other side of the fence, we were just sorry we couldn't be there on Monday morning to see the look on the custodians face when he discovered it. Needless to say, from that point on we always left a note on the gate for someone to let us know when it was going to be locked.

I had a few out-of-town visitors in March. The first visit came from my college roommate, Rick, the guy who had the patience and the misfortune of having to endure my rowdy late 60's antics during my many freshman years. He remembers them better than I do. Rick was in town on a college fund-raising trip and cut out an evening to get together. We had dinner at the "Pig and Whistle" restaurant in Hollywood, one of the hangouts of the stars of the Golden Age of film. It was both fun and melancholy. Fun in that we relived a lot of those insane days, still amazed that we survived; melancholy in that I was talking about a past life that I had lived without a care that was truly now gone.

On March 27, an old corporate friend, Mark, was in town and took me out to dinner for my 60th birthday. A year earlier on my 59th, I felt young. This year I felt every day my age. We went to a Greek restaurant and once again I tasted the food. It was then I realized that if I wanted to taste food, it should be Greek. To this day I have no clue why.

There were still bumps along the way. I discovered that State

Disability paperwork was being held up at the clinic and disability payments had stopped again, leaving a financial disaster. And there was the noise. The neighbors were relentless. I rarely had a sound night of sleep. But things were moving ahead and if all went well, I would soon be going back to work.

Unfortunately, all did not go well. Every time I would walk out of my building and into the sun, the now not-so-paralyzed side of my face would ball up in a tight muscle spasm. The same would happen in my sleep at night. I'd wake up in the morning with my mouth in a snarl. Whenever I ate or drank, my eye would close involuntarily. Whenever I laughed or yawned, the muscles in my neck would cramp up. I had hoped that it was just part of the nerve-regenerating process.

I shared my experiences with members of the Forum. Some members who had similar conditions, suggested it might be Synkinesis – something I had no clue what it was (neither does Spell-check apparently). In anything I had read about facial palsy exercises, there always seemed to be the warning, "watch out for Synkinesis." I had always assumed it was a temporary condition that would only delay my recovery since the explanation didn't go into its severity.

In early May, my doctor confirmed it. I had developed Synkinesis – the thing that would take two years for me to be about normal. When my facial nerves had regenerated, they had rewired wrong. Now signals from my brain to my eye were now going to my mouth and cheek and signals for my mouth and cheek were going to my eye. At least that's the way I understood it. He referred me to a physical therapist who dealt with facial and balance issues.

Things were getting real old real fast. It had been six long, confusing, irritating months since my surgery. Instead of being well on the road to recovery, I was falling deeper into a hole – a darkness where I began to wonder what else could happen to me that I hadn't being told. I didn't feel sorry for myself. I never asked "why me?" I shed no tears. I still had my faith. I was just angry – but I had no particular target for the anger.

CHAPTER FOUR

Nothing Gonna Keep Me Down

October 8, 2008

We did it. It wasn't pretty. The last three miles were just plain ugly. But less than a year after my surgery, with Britannia and her friend, Jasmin, I ran a Half Marathon. I hadn't given up.

It started not long after I got the news that I was now on a two-year road to recovery. On a cool, gray morning in early May, Britannia and I ran the Revlon Run for the Cure that we had so diligently trained for on the Long Beach tracks. It was a 5k run that we started on the streets of LA under a blast of confetti with about 30,000 other runners and walkers. We finished the race running through a tunnel and on to the field at USC's Coliseum three miles and 30 minutes later, the same tunnel where Marathoners had run through in the 1984 Olympics. We had run it in years past, but this year was special. Six months earlier I had brain tumor surgery. And we actually ran it faster than we had in past years.

Not long after that, I made a casual suggestion to Britannia. The summer before we had run the Peachtree Road Race in Atlanta, a 10K (for those of you who missed Metrics class like I did, that's a little over six miles). It was Britannia's first Peachtree and about my 20th. That started us on a dad-daughter running spree. My casual suggestion – since we had already run a 10K, why not try a Half-Marathon? (Note: don't make casual suggestions about something that isn't so casual). I had run them before and even a full Marathon, but not in quite some time. Britannia jumped on the idea and that started out an amazing summer.

Every Saturday morning that summer, I would walk six blocks through the deserted, early dawn, storefront streets of neighboring Koreatown to the subway that ran to downtown LA. There I caught a light-rail train that ran south through Watts, Compton and Long Beach. From Long Beach I would take a shuttle bus four miles south to Belmont Shore. Belmont Shore is a sleepy artist village of narrow streets populated with eclectic houses, condos, apartments, and a main street of sidewalk cafes, beach bars and boutiques. Britannia lived there. That's where we started.

Along the ocean by the sandy beaches and the Pacific Ocean, there is a concrete bike and walking path that runs from laidback Belmont Shore four miles north to the thriving city of Long Beach. It's a favorite of cyclists, runners, walkers, skateboarders, and drunken beach-bums who happened to stagger out on to it. That's the path the three of us would run every Saturday morning. We started out slow at shorter distances of three miles. But within months, Britannia, Jasmin and I were running up to 10 miles – two young California girls with their ponytails bouncing in the breeze and an old guy trying to put surgery and bad news behind him.

It was a busy summer; I wasn't going to let the bad news go ugly and I didn't want anger to consume what good there was. While all the running stuff was going on, I was trying to get my life back together. As soon as I found out my recovery was going to take two years, I marched my butt – well actually I stumbled my wonkyheaded self down to the local Social Security office to apply for Social Security Disability. I expected the worse, but found a very understanding staff. Folks on the Acoustic Neuroma forum had passed along the not so pleasant experiences they had encountered – some of them lasting over two years. My intake councilor, Mrs. Park, was understanding and compassionate. She was a bright spot in an otherwise grim existence.

Now I should probably mention something. I just wrote about running 10 miles. That obviously doesn't sound very disabled. Actually, with the balance issues that I had, there was no way that I could run by myself. If I tried to and took one off balance step because I had no focus, I would fall over, which I still occasionally did. I could do it, however with Britannia who was there to guide me. I just wanted to note that so I didn't lose anyone here who thought this jerk is scamming the system. Anyway, if this book becomes a best-seller (which I am hoping for), payments from Social Security would be discontinued until I reach retirement age.

Do your part to get Dave off Social Security and save the system. Encourage others to buy this book. (Have I no shame?)

The process started. There was a lengthy form that needed to be submitted along with the doctors' input. I knew I was messed up but would they see just how messed up I was. In mid-July, Social Security scheduled me for two tests to determine the level of my disability. The first test was administered by an ear doctor. I had heard that the offices that are contracted to perform the tests are looking for ways to disqualify applicants. That makes sense. I'm quite sure they see all sorts of cons and when they saw me walk into the office with a cane, I noticed a few smirks as they took me for a yet another fraud. When I told the doctor that I had had AN surgery, he realized I was totally deaf in one ear. When the audiologist gave me a hearing test, they had to realize that I was almost totally deaf, and for the most part without a hearing aid, I am.

The next test was a neurological exam. I really had no idea what to expect. Coupled with the balance issues there was a problem with disorientation – occasionally I would see things differently. Would they be able to determine that? I took the bus to a seedy area of town and found an even seedier clinic with boarded-up windows on the first floor of what looked to be an otherwise vacant four-story building. At one time the building seemed to be an attempt to bring some class to the neighborhood. Apparently the neighborhood won that struggle and the building now fit right in with all the no-name strip center, liquor store, street-corner food stand squalor. I pushed through the tinted glass, multi-lock door and into the waiting room. What I saw was jarring. It was a large room with buzzing overhead florescent lights and groaning in-room air conditioners. The mismatched chairs looked like a collection from the furniture section at a Goodwill center. It was gray and grim. But even more startling were the 30 or so patients. They were obviously poor. But even worse, they looked to be dead. Were it not for an occasional cough, I would take it for a morgue. I tried to blend in sitting on a metal folding chair and remaining as lifeless and pale as I possibly could.

Finally I was taken back to what could only be described as an interrogation room. It was as stark as the waiting room. The one window in the room had been painted black. Chips in the paint let tiny flecks of sunlight stream in. There was one metal desk, one metal chair, and one metal examination table. Nothing else. The only sign of life in the place was one fluorescent light buzzing overhead. It's partner was dead.

I waited. One hour. Two hours. My mind was slipping away. I tried to give my brain something to do. I tried to name all my teachers from Kindergarten through college – I couldn't remember my college Biology professor. I named all the Pittsburgh Pirates in the 1960 World Series – even naming the Yankees they were playing against. I made up stories. I stared. Then just as my brain was about to shut down and go into hibernation, she showed up at the door. She was the neurologist who would be getting a confession out of me. At least that was how it seemed.

There was some confusion at first about the seating arrangements since there was only one chair in the room and I was sitting on it. I offered it to her but she rolled in a chair from another room. I remember little about our conversation. She asked me a lot of questions. I answered honestly. She seemed to appreciate that. But what amazed me most was the physical test. She had me sit on the exam table and she banged my knee with a knee-jerk hammer. My knee didn't jerk. She tried again. No jerk. I think I was more surprised than she was. Up until that moment, I hadn't realized just how messed up I was. That was all there was to the exam. I left the clinic without a clue. How does one actually know whether they passed or failed a neurological exam?

I rolled through August with no communications from Social Security. Folks on the Acoustic Neuroma forum with Social Security experience said it could take years to hear anything and even then it was a denial that would be tied up in court and maybe eventually granted. I figured by that time I would be living in a cardboard box on Skidrow.

Then in early September, it happened. I began to get obscure messages on my Social Security account page. One such message read that I shouldn't open the "Check My Benefits" page until I received my notification letter. Notification Letter! I immediately hopped on the Forum asking what a Notification Letter meant. There were several other Forum members who had received Social Security Disability – but not without intense, protracted legal haggling. None of them could recall an approval letter so soon in the process, but all were in agreement – it sounded like The Letter.

I soon received notification that I would receive a letter on or about September 9. That day I paced, I prayed, I paced some more. I made a 1,000 or so trips to the mailbox. Finally, at 3:12 PM PDT, I opened the mailbox and it was there. I tore the envelop open and read. I was approved. The benefits would begin in October. I felt incredible relief. It was the best news I had received since the mess started a year earlier. Now if I needed to wait two years for my face to be "about normal" and my balance to improve to non-stagger, I could afford to do it – not extravagantly, but enough to keep a roof over my head and food on my plate.

There were some other highlights that summer. In addition to the Saturday runs in Long Beach, I was getting out more often with the help of friends. I'd go over to Cindy's place in Hollywood to grill steaks. We'd watch Sun's basketball games and she introduced me to *American Idol*. I've never forgiven her. James and I continued to hike and on July 4th, he and his wife Tracie invited me over to their place in Burbank for a cook out. It was a good break from so much of the sameness.

I found what I thought was going to be a big money-maker that I could do at the comfort of my desk. In my early career, I had a background in graphic design and copywriting. In the 35 years since, the methods had changed but the basics hadn't. So I thought I would put them to use designing T-shirts and Gifts on Café Press. Being a Christian and an athlete, I decided I would combine the two and create a series of shirts and gifts using Paul's advice to the Philippians: "I can do all things through Him who strengthens me." It's a good piece of inspiration to Christian athletes. Only I may need to work a little harder when it comes to selling shirts and gifts. I sold one T-shirt in two years. So much for my new career. Here's an example of one for runners.

www.cafepress.com/BritanniaK2.

Another moment that transformed my post-surgery life came in August. I had been helping a member of the Acoustic Neuroma forum find a Southern California post-surgery getaway. Kathleen was from Colorado and was having her surgery through the same clinic that I had. Following surgery, patients are required to stay within range of LA for two weeks for follow-up visits and to insure a trouble-free recovery. I knew the SoCal haunts that would make the recovery as pleasant as it could be and gave Kathleen my recommendations. In the process, I noticed that I had an eye-doctor appointment a few days after her surgery. I suggested that it might be fun to meet in St. Vincent's cafeteria after my eye appointment. Nancy, another Acoustic Neuroma forum member, was having her pre-surgery physical that day and joined in.

It was an incredible experience; they were the first ANers I had met nearly nine months post-surgery. Kathleen was in great shape – I wasn't anywhere near as good as she was that soon after surgery. She did admit to being tired which is a common symptom among posties.

Nancy, a beautiful lady with a compassionate heart and an awesome smile, was full of questions and a little apprehension. Her surgery was the next day. She came through with colors – no issues.

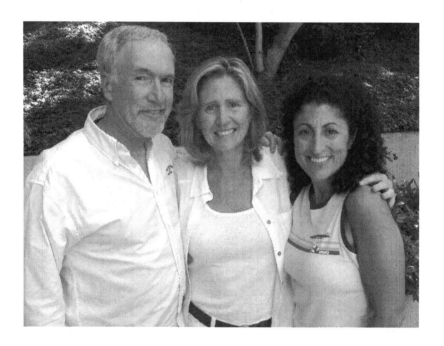

My first ANer meeting with Kathleen and Nancy. August 5, 2008

Little did we know it at the time, but that get together with the three of us in St. Vincent's cafeteria by the shaded courtyard, started a tradition that is carried on to this day. Not long after Nancy's surgery and recovery, she noticed on the ANA Forum that Cheri, a young mom from Texas, was on her way to the clinic for surgery. Since Nancy felt like it had done so much to help build her confidence to meet with me and Kathleen, she felt like we might be able to help others. So, on a warm day in late September, Nancy, Lainie – a fellow ANer from Los Angeles that Nancy and I had just befriended, and I dropped into to the hospital cafeteria to meet Cheri and her husband, Mike. They were a wonderful couple, full of life with a great sense of humor. To this day, I consider them two of my best friends.

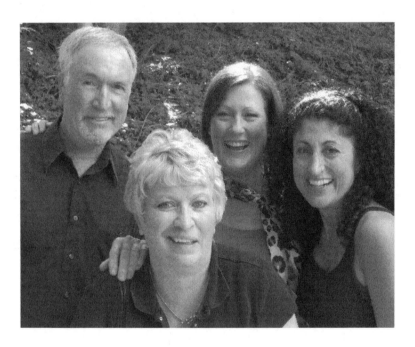

Me, Lainie, Cheri, and Nancy in St Vincent's Courtyard

Lainie, a Brit with a wicked wit and a way of putting things in a proper perspective, fit right in and was adding her spin on the great

AN adventure. Lainie too had the facial paralysis from her surgery that I had. It was comforting in an odd way to realize that I was not alone and to see that another who was so endowed with palsy could carry on a normal life. I also realized that it was probably a lot more devastating to a woman than to some old guy. I've since come across more women who have been affected by the facial palsy and Synkinesis. They've been an inspiration to me in the way that they've dealt with it. Of course that may come off a bit sexist as if saying women are more vain than men. I've been married one too many times to let that go unmentioned. It just seems that men get a pass on things like wrinkles and issues like facial palsy. Women don't.

The three of us had a busy fall of 2008. As we soon learned, patients were scheduling their surgeries before the year end because their deductibles had been met with tests and all the stuff that lead up to the big show. They came from all over the United States and as far away as Singapore and The Netherlands. Nearly every week we'd find ourselves in St. Vincent's cafeteria. A few times we met at the Grove, a shopping/restaurant complex that was a favorite of the stars on the Hollywood side of the hill. Eventually, we began to take on roles. Nancy, the caring and informative one (she understood the medical stuff); Lainie and I the color commentators adding humor to an otherwise bleak situation – sort of the Acoustic Neuroma version of Monday Night Football announcers.

Spending time with others before their surgeries meant a lot to me. I went into my surgery unprepared with no fellow ANer's there for support. I knew how un-nerving, confusing and lonely that was – it was the least I could do to be there for others.

Not long after I got the "about normal" news from my doctor, I began the long road of physical therapy to become "about normal." My physical therapist was one of a few who specialized in facial reanimation (she worked with Mary Jo Buttafuco) and palsy patients as well as working with patients with balance issues – issues like randomly falling over. Unfortunately her office was in Orange County, 40 miles south of where I lived and I couldn't drive. So with the help of my friend, Linda, I would make my way to Garden Grove every two weeks for physical therapy.

The first leg of the trip was a six block stagger through Koreatown to the subway that took me downtown to connect to the Blueline train that ran from LA to Long Beach through the industrial sprawl of South Central LA. In Long Beach I'd meet Linda who would drive me through the beach towns and areas that fed Disneyland to my PT's office in Garden Grove just a block from Robert Schuller's Crystal Cathedral. It's hard to put a finger on the main difference between Los Angeles and Orange County, but they are different. I guess it could be summed up in two words "planned development" – in the OC some thought was given as opposed to LA where random chaos ruled. The change of scenery and fresh air was a nice break.

PT wasn't so pleasant. I don't know what gave me the impression that something that would undo all the evil stuff that had happened to me would be fun. The office was a spacious and modern place set in a charming, shaded office park with white wooden steps running to the second level. It masked the torture waiting within its walls.

The first macabre machine I faced was the evil balance box, or in my case, the unbalance box. The three-walled machine was designed to test one's balance and relay the information to a computer which analyzed it. I learned there were three components of balance. They have scientific names for them but since I avoid using scientific terms, here's what they are in my terms: sensory leg strength, eye coordination and the inner ear balance nerve of which I had only one left. That lonely nerve was supposed to be compensating for the nerve on the other side that had been removed during surgery. The machine tested these three functions independently to pinpoint where the balance issues lie.

First up was the leg sensory test. I nailed that. I'm guessing it had to do something with all the pre and post surgery running and hiking I had been doing. The vision test was next. While not as good as the leg stability test, it was still nearly acceptable. The inner ear test was a disaster. With my eyes closed, the machine suddenly transformed itself into a moving funhouse floor lunging and tossing me in every direction. The computer scored several falls. In other words, in a normal walking situation if I didn't have strong legs and reasonably good vision, I would fall over. Earlier in the year, as I was particularly tired and my legs were a bit weak, I did just that – fell over in the street like a stumbling drunk. It wasn't pretty as I flailed around trying to regain my balance before landing in a humiliated heap.

My PT gave me balance exercises to do at home. I'd stand in a corner on a cushion with my eyes focused on an object. I'd do the drunk test heal-toe walk. I'd try to stand on one leg. I suppose they worked temporarily. But as soon as my sole balance nerve felt neglected, it got all pouty and sulked off into a corner. A few years later I would discover that there was another issue that caused my balance to be off that no one had considered – and if they did, they failed to mention it. For some reason, I believe my medical providers felt like I could only handle information in small doses – as though they didn't want to overwhelm me with facts – facts like, "You're messed up, Bud."

Next up on the PT torture roster after the balance training was the face-mangling. Deep-tissue massage on the body is intense enough. Deep-tissue massage on the face is downright pain ugly. The massage is designed to loosen up the tight muscles caused by paralysis and synkinesis so they could function "almost normally" and prevent the mis-wired nerves from getting too weird. It involved all this rubbing and pulling and squeezing and beating – even a massage of my cheek from the inside of my mouth. It worked to an extent. That summer I was finally able to sip liquids through a straw and eat without most of the food falling from the corner of my mouth. I achieved a new level of sociability. I could almost eat comfortably in public without being an embarrassment to myself and those around me. The PT gave me face-mangling exercises to do at home – although I wasn't quite as brutal as the PT was.

As gruesome as the PT sessions were, I continued making my regular trips to Garden Grove. I made it a social outing. After my PT sessions, Linda and I would join friends for lunch at ocean-side restaurants. It was a welcomed break from an otherwise tedious and solitary life. Unfortunately the hour-long train ride coming back from Long Beach to LA past miles of urban grey junkyards and auto body shops was a somber reminder of the dour solitary life I was dealing with.

There was one major disappointment during the summer. Of all things, it had to do with my church. I go to a contemporary Christian church called Oasis – not particularly big by Saddleback standards –

but it had a strong gathering of young people from throughout the Hollywood area. Due to its size and the fact that many of the tithers are struggling actors and musicians, the church relies heavily on volunteer efforts. So I felt like since I had the time, I could do some volunteer work in the church office during the week. In that I had an extensive marketing background, I believed I could assist with advice on their membership recruitment and community outreach. I contacted Jeff, the associate pastor who had followed my recovery and volunteered my time starting one day a week.

Apparently I hadn't communicated my marketing background well enough or maybe they just didn't want members meddling in their marketing plans. I was asked to do research on seminars. Of course I was anxious to serve in whatever capacity and eagerly agreed by throwing myself into the project. While I am fairly proficient in "googling" my way around the internet, I was working on an unfamiliar computer and system. After about an hour of research, my brain began to act up and disorientation began to set in. Up to that point, I hadn't focused on anything particular that required a great deal of concentration. My head started spinning but I kept on researching along. After about three hours I had to give up and go home.

I gave it another shot a week later. My assignment was to merge and purge church records. It wasn't any better. I could barely sit upright in a chair and when I stood to greet people who stopped by to say hi, I staggered to my feet and weaved back and forth like a drunk – which I'm sure they thought I was – not something particularly endearing in a church office. I couldn't do it. I wanted to be productive. I wanted to contribute my time. But I just couldn't handle it. I felt useless. At the same time I realized that I wouldn't be able to deal in a normal work environment where I would be expected to produce. My options for returning as a productive member of society were narrowing. It was one of those nasty little surprises that I hadn't counted on. The ride home that day on the subway from the Valley to Hollywood was bleak.

There was good stuff. The SAG Foundation was an incredible bright spot in my life that summer. The Foundation, affiliated with the Screen Actors Guild, is an organization that provides services and resources to the acting community like workshops, training, children's literacy programs, and college scholarships. It is funded by voluntary contributions from actors to assist other actors. One of the areas of assistance is the emergency financial fund. Actors in financial need can apply for, and receive assistance to meet the most basic needs such as rent, car payments, and medical bills. I realize of course that most people see actors as financially well-off. There are the stars who do live lavish life-styles. But the working class actor struggles. Roles are often random. And what was a good month can suddenly become a string of bad months. With all the unanticipated medical bills I had accumulated post-surgery and the difficulty of living on State Disability, I had become overwhelmed with medical expenses – and those bills needed to be paid to continue my physical therapy. I applied to the Foundation and I was approved. The Foundation covered the bills that I had racked up. Not only did they do that, but when my Screen Actors Guild health insurance expired in October because I hadn't been able to act, the Foundation also covered my COBRA payments for the next 18 months of eligibility. Stacey, the emergency fund coordinator, and the Foundation were a blessing.

In spite of the balance issues, face palsy, hearing loss, disorientation and all the other annoying stuff crowding my life, on a chilly morning in early October, I ended that summer by running the Long Beach Half-Marathon, ten months after my surgery when I still believed that I had a chance for a full recovery. I met Britannia and Jasmin before dawn to make our way to the race start along the ocean on the Grand Prix course in downtown Long Beach. We joined 20,000 or so other runners for the 13-mile run (some braver souls were running a full Marathon). The course route took us across a long bridge to the Queen Mary side of the bay. My knee was painful. It felt like bone grinding on bone (as I later discovered, I had developed arthritis). But I gamely gimped along. The weather was perfect, sunny and crisp. We never saw the Queen Mary – something that's a bit hard to miss. Instead we wound our way through a maze of faceless hotels, apartments and condos. Eventually we stumbled our way back across the bridge to Long Beach – the halfway point where we miscalculated that we were two or three days off pace. Then we ran down the bike path along the ocean where we had trained all those summer Saturday mornings to Belmont Shore, the tree-shaded ocean-side village where we made a turn to head back to the finish.

Those last three miles, as we passed parks where Frisbee-throwing people and their dogs frolicked carefree and ocean-front condos where residents smugly sipped their morning Maitais, were just ugly. As anyone who has run a Marathon or a Half knows, the last part of the race goes from doomed to worse. We all had some ailment. I had a bad knee. Britannia had a bad shin. Jasmin was in a bad mood. Walkers were walking faster than we were running. But at two hours and 30 minutes we crossed the finish line, well back in the pack – well actually, the pack had long before crossed the line – we were stragglers. I couldn't have done it without my daughter running by my side, guiding me, steadying me and encouraging me. It would be the last race for some time to come. I had done some damage to my knee and with the newly discovered arthritis, it made it harder to recover. Later that day, Britannia and I had a celebration dinner at Gladstones by the ocean just blocks from where we had started the race in the morning. It was an incredible end to an amazing summer.

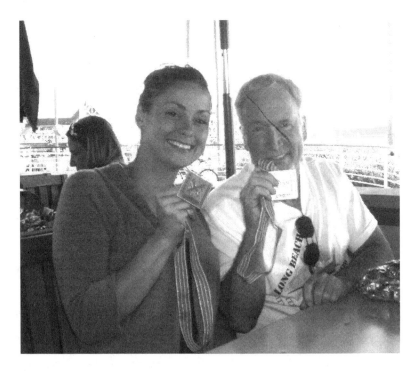

The Half Marathon Celebration Dinner

CHAPTER FIVE

The Last Smile

September 15, 2009

"Never!" That's all I heard. She said it another way as she mangled my face. Here's what she said, sort of nonchalantly, the way they all seem to do when they break the bad news. Like saying things nonchalantly makes them not so bad.

"Know that email you forwarded to me? It's true. Your face will never recover. We can only manage it with therapy."

So let me get this straight. That two months that turned into a year that turned into two years is now never? Never! My face will be permanently deformed? Somewhere early in the process, I think it would have been a good idea to let me in on the secret that I was messed up and that's the way it is and will be, "so suck it up, Bucko" instead of trading reality for false hopes.

My second year post-surgery was as strangely adventurous as was my first. Soon after the Half-Marathon, I moved to the top floor of my building to a serene place with an expansive view of snow-covered mountains to the left and the downtown LA skyline to the right and mercifully away from the noisy neighbors. I discovered a new-found peace for my recovery. I also discovered that my 15-year-old cat, Yikes, had diabetes which threw a curveball into our lives. We were now on an insulin shot time schedule. I could now be no more than 12-hours from home to give her the shots. It put me on a short leash. The two of us settled into our new existence.

Not long after that, I started my own series of shots. Botox. Botox is of course the de rigor for Hollywood's sagging faces – the promise of perpetual superficial youth in a syringe. My treatments weren't for that purpose. The Synkinesis in my face was causing muscles to do weird things. The intended blink of an eye would cause a snarl of the lip. Carefully targeted Botox injections would freeze muscles that were causing the involuntary reactions allowing normal muscle movements a chance to recover independently. At least that's the way I understood it.

I never liked needles. They are unnecessary angry little things. There are plenty of other holes in the body like the mouth or the nose without going out and making new ones. But as I was soon to discover, a needle in the arm was nothing compared to a needle in the face. It's insane – and what is even more insane, people do it voluntarily.

My doctor held a Botox clinic monthly. Apparently I wasn't alone. There were others with "about normal" faces. It was about a year to the day after my surgery when I met with him for my first round of Botox injections. He had me make face movements so he could ID the rogue muscles. Once he had the bad guys figured out, he drew out that grim steel syringe. The first injection was in my eyebrow. He warned me that it would sting a little. A little?!?! This guy was the master of understatements. That little sting was more like ice-pick jabbed in my eye. It hurt – a lot! There's little pain that can cause me to cry, but I had man tears, not the kind that roll down your cheek but the ones that well-up in your eyes that you hope no one notices.

That was it! No more shots. But before I could run away he nailed me with the second shot, this time in my lower eyelid – even more painful than the first. Then one in the corner of my mouth. And to conclude the diabolical event, the grand finale – three shots in the neck. I struggled to keep my man tears in my eyes as I questioned the sanity of anyone who would do this voluntarily. That day I learned the depth of vanity.

The session was over. I couldn't tell the difference – it would take several weeks. To this day, after about five sessions, I'm still unsure about the effectiveness. But in all fairness, it's difficult to measure progress or the lack of it on a day-to-day basis. I'm better than I was three years ago, but am I better or worse than I was a year ago or even a week ago? It all seems the same – pre-surgery life compared to post-surgery life. In one I was normal. The other I am not normal.

About the same time as the Botox ordeal, I had a fleeting moment of "fame." I wanted to tell my story. I had believed that I was nearing the recovery finish line and I felt as though I could pass along "all" my wisdom to rookie ANers. After all, I was a very seasoned, one-year vet. Little did I know what else was in store.

So with all the naiveté I could muster, I told my story to that point. I wrote an article for the Acoustic Neuroma Association's quarterly newsletter. It was published in the September 2008 edition under a column called "Voyages." I felt productive for a change. This book is to a degree based on that article. When I wrote it I was filled with fearless bravado fully expecting to make a full recovery not knowing the lurking truth. Today I know the truth. The bravado is gone.

The second moment under the lights came with an article published in the SAG Magazine, a national publication for members of the Screen Actors Guild. The magazine was planning to do a feature on the Screen Actors Guild Foundation; the Foundation that had supported me by financially assisting me with medical bills and insurance premiums.

Stacey, the emergency funds coordinator at the time, asked me if I would be willing to let them do a feature article on my recovery and my support from the Foundation. The spotlight – in front of my peers – on stage again? Why of course I'd be willing. I'd be returning to work someday and I'd have an edge up on notability with casting directors.

"Say, aren't you that brain tumor guy? Welcome back," they'd gush. "May I be the first to offer you a big part in a movie with an obscenely large contract?" (Or at least I think that's the way my addled brain was working at the time. This actually would be the farthest thing from the truth in the acting business). But most importantly, it would give me the opportunity to publicly thank the Foundation for their support.

So on November 5th, I met the writer from SAG Magazine at my physical therapist's office to do a photo shoot. We did a series of shots on each of the torture machines. About a month later, the magazine came out. I was a national two-page spread special; one page a bunch of pictures from the PT's office, the other an article on my surgery and recovery. To this day, other actors I work with comment on that article. Until that point, many of them had thought I had disappeared. I did too.

I spent a peaceful Thanksgiving and Christmas with Britannia at her place on the ocean. As usual there was some confusion over cooking and roasting times but a festive time was had by all – probably a little too festive which is what led to the cooking confusion. Fortunately no one landed in the hospital.

During the holidays I also discovered Facebook and in the process, discovered more stuff about friends that I didn't need to know. It still amazes me what foolish and odd things normally sane people will say behind the guise of anonymity while hunched over a computer keyboard in various stages of dress and grooming.

In the beginning, I was flooded by friend requests by semi-famous people. I was flattered. Me? You want me to be your friend? Why of course. We'll be buddies – have coffee, do the club circuit, ride up the coast for an afternoon of wild and crazy times. And think of the fun I would have name-dropping and how impressed my lesser friends will be when they see my "star" buddies and buddets on my Facebook friends list. It was later for me (as it usually is) that I discovered that amassing a sea of "friends" is a means of self-promotion for struggling nobodies and that I was just another name on the list. I was so distraught that I briefly flirted with the notion of taking a razor blade to my computer cord. Instead I had a grand old party deleting them all. That showed them.

At the same time, I connected with a lot of lost "real" acquaintances. Apparently they weren't lost. They actually had a life too and didn't just put their lives on hold frozen in the past for my convenience. And finally, I discovered dumb. Why anyone would want to parade their narrow-minded *opinions* as though they were irrefutable fact and do it with guileless pride is quite beyond me. They need a brain tumor to put things in perspective. Just give me the family news, the baby that took its first steps, vacation fun, great meals, a race that was run, friends that got together, a grandma celebrating her 90th birthday, cheering for a team and a country's freedom, funny stuff and prayer requests – and if absolutely necessary, the "just saying" thoughts. The rest of it doesn't count for much in the long run.

As 2009 started, I was back to visiting AN patients with Nancy and Lainie. In January, we had an unexpected treat. Marci, an AN survivor we met on the Forum was in town with The Oberlin College Symphony Orchestra. She was the Associate Dean for the Conservatory of Music. The orchestra was playing at the Disney Concert Hall in downtown LA – a very elegant place – the Concert Hall, not downtown LA. Marci invited us to a Sunday matinee performance. It was a classy event – the first time I had worn dress-em-up shoes instead of running shoes in the year since my surgery. I had been raised on classical music and while I wasn't familiar with the selections, I could appreciate them and the orchestra as being outstanding – and a nice break from all the football games I had been immersed in on television. It was an incredible to start the year – quite a contrast to my grim existence a year earlier.

Shannon

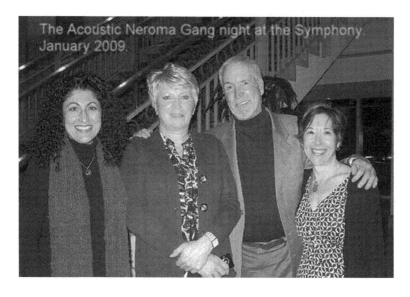

Nancy, Lainie, me, and Marci at the Symphony

Throughout the early part of the year, we met with more amazing people who were headed into surgery. They were beautiful, fun, positive and they all had one thing in common – they were brave. But there was one who stood out. Her name was Beth, a pretty 24-year-old from Louisiana. Beth's first surgery had gone bad. I don't remember the particulars but in addition to having a stroke, she had permanently lost all her hearing as well as having the facial palsy that many of us have. She was in town to have yet another surgery. I don't recall off-hand what it was for; there were so many and they all had technical names. I asked her to give me a list so I could try to explain what she had been through. And I felt like my one surgery was a difficult thing to handle! Here's the list of the surgeries and procedures that she had to deal with in her own words:

- *July 2006 VP shunt placement* *
- *Sept 2006 laminectomy (spinal neurofibroma resection)*
- *Oct 2006 - PEG tube placement*
- *Oct 2006 right vestibular schwannoma (vs) resection (retrosigmoid approach)* *
- *Feb 2007 left vs resection (retrosigmoid approach)* *
- *Aug 2007 gold weight implant in left eyelid*
- *Sept 2007 tarsorraphy (sp?) of left eyelid*
- *Jan 2008 left vs resection (translabrynthine approach) and abi (auditory brainstem implant) placement* *
- *March 2008 CN 7-12 anastamosis, left side* *
- *April 2008 thoracotomy (chest wall neurofibroma resection)*
- *Sept 2008 lap cholecystectomy*
- *Nov 2008 left tarsal tunnel neurofibroma resection*
- *March 2009 right vs resection (translabrynthine approach) and abi placement* *
- *March 2009 gold weight placement in right eyelid*
- *April 2009 hematoma (llq of abdomen, secondary to translab sx) evacuation*
- *Jan 2010 - meningioma in occipital lobe of the brain ressected* *

Ok so those are the sx's (I had a list so I just copied and pasted). The ones with the stars after them are brain surgeries. The spinal surgery and the thoracotomy were also really big surgeries to remove tumors. I couldn't walk for the first 8 mos. once it all started b/c after the shunt was placed to relieve the hydrocephaly the AN's grew so big they were sqashing my brainstem (literally). I was like a baby. I couldn't eat, chew, dress myself, do anything with my hands, walk, sit up, use the restroom, write, I couldn't do anything. I had to have a feeding tube placed in my stomach. But I got better after the 2nd AN sx.

I don't know what my prognosis is. No one has ever told me. At first my main neurosurgeon said I would die in surgery when he was getting ready to remove the tumors for the first time. But I'm a soldier (haha) and I'm tough and I don't think I will die any time soon. Although I have read that the life expectancy for nf2 is 40-50 yrs, but that's just an avg. Next time we come to LA I will ask the doctors there about it, b/c my doctors here really don't know. They don't have another nf2 patient.

She and her devoted husband and a devout Christian, Joseph, were in town for yet another surgery for Beth. We had dinner with them that night at a California Pizza Kitchen in downtown LA. Beth was pretty good at reading lips. She had a problem reading mine because my lips didn't move well. Whatever she didn't understand, Joseph would sign to her and she would respond as best she could without hearing the sound of her own words. As I discovered, she was bright, charming, and a bit of a teaser. I remember how blessed I felt to meet someone so young with so much faith and determination. She could have been mad at the world for being robbed of a normal life but she pushed ahead, her spirit bright and unbeatable.

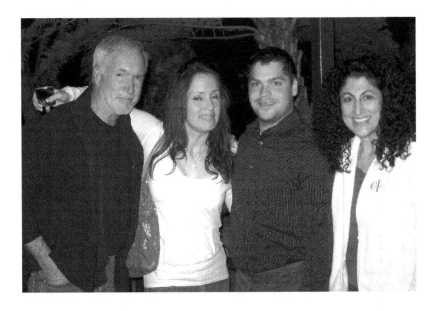

Me, Beth, Joseph and Nancy outside St Vincent's 3/1/09

Beth gave me new-found inspiration to keep moving ahead and refuse to give up. I did just that. Since the completion of the Half-Marathon, I had fallen into a funk. It wasn't a feel sorry for me morose kind of thing – more like an aimless, uninspired, unmotivated, goal-less, go through the motions sort of existence. I really wasn't taking anything on much more than getting up in the morning, feeding myself, feeding the cat, and going to sleep at night. With my Beth-recharged faith, I started back on a path of renewed recovery. I rejoined the gym that I hadn't been to since a month before my surgery. Sure I had to take the bus to get there. Sure I stumbled around a lot. Sure it reminded me of where I my physical well-being had once been. But I went back. To this day, I continue to go.

In the spring, I started joining Britannia on her canvassing ventures. She works for a mall management and development company and is responsible for leasing space in the two malls she is assigned. She's always looking for new concepts and companies that might fit her leasing opportunities. To find retail matches, she picks an area of town that is similar to the areas surrounding her malls. She then visits retail operations in those malls and "encourages" them to seek new pastures – like her malls. While she doesn't necessarily need it, I tag along providing my marketing and merchandising input that I gained in years of corporate marketing. Actually, I think she just invited me along to get me out of the house. But it did make me feel productive.

In March, I chanced kayaking – something that I was very adept at pre-surgery. Post surgery it would be a challenge since good balance is critical and I was a bit short on the balance meter. One crisp, early morning, when the mist still drifted above the water, Britannia, Jasmin and I set out on a kayak adventure around Naples south of Long Beach.

Naples is a yacht-club community with inter-locking canals, the perfect place to try out my questionable balance on still water. The only problem was that Naples was on the other side of a wide choppy bay from the kayak launch beach. I had to make that crossing first.

So with life jacket tightly secured (I wasn't sure if I could swim post-surgery), I slid my kayak off the sand and into the water. In the past, I would have gracefully slipped onboard. No such luck this time. I looked like a floundering fish that had just plopped out of the water. I was praying that no one had seen it. In reality, while I didn't want to actually look up, I was sure that everyone on the beach was watching me and a TV News crew who had just happened to be there taping a segment for the evening news, caught me in the act. This of course was doomed to be broadcast with some anchor making snarky remarks about some clumsy tourist – the life jacket being the giveaway. I didn't have to look to see it. It's just one of those things that you know instinctively. I awkwardly regained some of my composure and began to paddle.

By now, the two girls were far ahead of me in the rough, open water. I paddled harder. As I did, I noticed something. My balance, or lack of it, was not an issue. It was a thrill churning hard through the waves in the bay with the wind spray blowing in my face. Before long I caught up with the girls. We made it across the bay and spent a leisurely morning paddling through the canals checking out Naple's exotic houses and massive yachts. The old guy was keeping up – and staying up. Of course I was reminded of my balance when we landed our kayaks on the beach. If getting in was awkward, getting out was a disaster as I unceremoniously fell backward on my butt in the shallows of the water's edge – much to the amusement of the girls and the kayak rental guys.

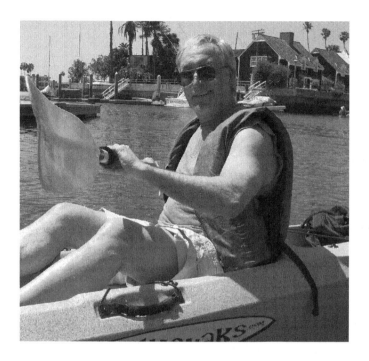

The Great Kayak Adventure

That spring, Britannia had been on a tear to learn every sport that guys played. The thinking being that if she met a guy who was interested in a particular sport she would be able to join him, giving her an advantage over any potential competition. One sport that she wanted to learn was music to my ears. Golf. Never did I imagine that my daughter would take up a sport that I loved -- although I shouldn't have been surprised – we did run together and play basketball.

I had played at golf since I was eight when my grandfather taught me to play on a ragged driving range in Cleveland. At one time in my life I was a four handicap. Over years of neglect, I had managed to whittle it down to a 20. (For those who don't know golf, this isn't a good thing). And living in Los Angeles didn't help my game where landing a tee-time at a sane hour is like winning the lottery and paying for the round takes the lottery winnings. But I still loved the game.

So on a gray, cool morning, I wrapped a few clubs together in mailing paper and taped them up and headed down to Long Beach. Why? A bag of clubs wouldn't have cut it on the Blue Line train which the local gangs use to shuttle between Watts and Compton. I mean really, some dorky white guy sitting on a light rail train with bag of golf clubs – I would have been laughed off – probably without my clubs. I might as well have been wearing knickers with a tam on my head.

Britannia borrowed a set of clubs from a friend. We headed over to the Long Beach Municipal Golf Course – a very good course for a public one – but the driving range tees were a bit of an after-thought. The tees were terraced down a slope, four tees to each terrace with a tall growth of shrubs and trees between each leaving us some privacy – unlike the public spectacle I made boarding the kayak a few weeks earlier. I was concerned, of course, that my balance would be an issue. And while I could play golf, I was never much good at describing the 100 or so individual movement in a golf swing that had become natural over time. I wasn't sure how well I would be able to instruct Britannia on those intricacies. That tee privacy was probably a good thing.

I hadn't played golf in about four years. To be safe, I started out with an iron. Not so safe. I topped the ball and watched in chagrin as it rolled ten feet in front of the tee. Britannia missed her first shot. Off to an ugly start. Then I got off a solid second shot – and realized that my balance wasn't really bothering me. Before long I was easily landing shots on the greens out in the driving range 180 yards away. I started paying more attention to Britannia. She is tall, strong and athletic and usually takes to a sport with little effort. But golf is a little more complex and as I feared, I wasn't the best teacher. But with the little help I gave her and with her own determination, she was soon hitting strong shots 100 yards out – a little to the left – but strong.

Several weeks later on a June-gloomy Father's Day at the Heartwell Par Three course where Tiger Woods learned to play, Britannia and I played nine holes. She beat me. It didn't matter. I was playing golf again and I taught my daughter to play golf well enough to beat me. We both won.

Physical Therapy took another odd turn that summer. My Physical Therapist had been selected to administer a balance training study called The BrainPort. According to the developer of the BrainPort: "The BrainPort balance devise is an investigational devise designed for training patients with balance deficits due to chronic vestibular disorders. The device provides information about the head position through electrotacile stimulation of the tongue. During training sessions, the patient places the electrode array on the tip of the tongue and........zzz

zzzzzzzzzzzzzzzzzzzzzzzzzzzzzzzzzzzzzzzzzzzzzzzzzzzzzzzzzzzzzzzzzzzz
zzzzzzzzzzzzzzzzzzzzzzzzzzzzzzzzzzzzzzzzzzzzzzzzzzzzzzzzzzzzzzzzzzzz
zzzzzzzzzzzzzzzzzzzzzzzzzzzzzzzzzzzzzzzzzzzzzzzzzzzzzzzzzzzzzzzzzzzz
zzzzzzzzzzzzzzzzzzzzzzzzzzzzzzzzzzzzzzzzz

So sorry. I drifted off there for a moment. It's that techno-algebra stuff. Here's what I can tell you about this. There's a magic box (since I can't quite grasp the concept of computer chips, the only logical explanation is that it's magic) you wear around your neck on a strap. A flat metal cable runs from the box to a sensor pad that you place on your tongue. Electric stimulation signals are sent back and forth between your brain and the box telling your brain when you're messing up on balance so your brain can fix things because you're too messed up to figure it out. At least that's what I, the lab rat, understood.

In order to qualify for the test, I had to go through a test in the PT's crazy balance machine – failed that. An in-office balance gait thing. Failed that. And an ENG. Now somewhere along the line one would think an individual of above average intelligence would look up ENG. I must be the dumbest clump in the universe. ENG? Sure, I'll do that. Couldn't be any worse than an MRI. Yes it could.

The technician was smiling as I entered the room – as usual. Why don't they just say "you're going to hate this," and go about their business? Most of the test is just tedious. I was strapped on a table (an omen of bad things to come), goggles were placed over my eyes and I was told that I needed to keep my eyes open and follow a blinking red light. Not too hard, although keeping my eyes open was a bit of a nuisance. Next she squirted water in my ear and the table began to move around. Annoying but tolerable. Then she excused herself to get "the ice water." I believe she went to the Arctic to get it. When she returned, she informed me that she would be shooting "the ice water" in my ear and that "it may be a little uncomfortable". By now, I had come to realize those words meant "run away while you can." I believe I tried to get up but I was strapped down to the table. They must have had other escapees in the past. She placed the water gun to my ear and shot. I don't remember if I screamed out loud, but I screamed somewhere. That was no ordinary ice water. If I had to guess, I would say it was about the temperature of liquid nitrogen. It was like an icicle being stabbed into my head. I closed my eyes and tensed in pain. She told me to open my eyes. I wanted to tell her something else. Then the table began to roll upside down. My thoughts drifted back to better times, like having brain surgery or getting Botox needles jabbed in my neck. As it always does, after an hour, the torture came to an end. Later my doctor would give me the results of the test; my vestibular system wasn't functioning properly. Pardon me. I stumble around like a drunk and you needed a test to prove my vestibular system was out of service? Fortunately, that was the last test. I qualified to be a BrainPort lab rat.

Like everything in my new brain tumor world, I didn't know what I was getting into. But I was tired of stumbling and weaving around and would try anything to get better. The test was to begin with a three-day training program at my PT's office in Garden Grove. For various reasons, rides from Linda were a thing of the past. So I would get up at dawn and wobble four blocks to the Metro subway that I took to Union Station. There I would catch Amtrak to Angel's baseball stadium. I'd like to mention that while Amtrak rarely made it to it's destination on time, it was a very comfortable ride – quite unlike the butt-numbing rides on the Los Angeles Light Rail trains. From Angel's Stadium I would walk a half mile to an intersection where I caught a bus to a retail-entertainment complex called The Block where I walked the remaining half mile to the PT's office to stand in a corner on a cushion with my eyes closed with this weird thing hanging around my neck and an electronic pad on my tongue for 20 minutes.

Then came the four-hour break when I was kicked out of the PTs office left on my own to kill time. A truly mind-numbing experience. Most people were close enough to the office that they could drive home for the break. I was 40 miles and several bus and train rides from home. I sat at The Block and stared a lot. It was summer and it was hot. I moved to a nearby hotel lobby where I pretended to be a guest for three hours. Then back to the PTs office to stand on a cushion in a corner with my eyes closed (I peaked once to make sure the test administrator wasn't laughing at me) with my buddy the Brainport leashed around my neck for another 20 minutes. I repeated that routine for a grueling three days before I launched into the program at home for the next eight weeks. Twice a day I'd stand on a cushion in a corner with my eyes closed with this thing strapped around my neck for 20 minutes. My cat stared at me as though I had lost my mind. About halfway into it, I too began to question my sanity. I meticulously recorded my activities in a daily log.

August 21, Day 40 of this madness. Stood in the corner for 20 minutes with my eyes closed this morning. Peeked once. Maybe twice. Moved my feet an inch closer together. Reality is slowly slipping away. Stood in the corner for 20 minutes with my eyes closed this evening. I think I heard the Brainport box talking. Or maybe it was the cat talking. Maybe they were talking to each other. I hope no one really reads this stuff. I think I need a drink.

It was tedious. And it appeared to be fruitless. But I really wanted my balance back.

There were two groups in the test. I may have been in the not so successful group. (Update: Recently I learned that the test was inconclusive, something the FDA doesn't like to hear). I do know that my balance is still a mess. And what I've read recently, because my brain has accepted vision and the legs as a satisfactory method of balance, my vestibular system may never be corrected.

I had better news that summer – two visits from some wonderful friends. The first was from my Christian brother, Steve. Steve and I had met on a movie set 12 years earlier and became instant friends sharing a bond in our Christian faith. Several years after we met, Steve threw in the towel on acting (a wise move) and he and his wife, Susan moved to Atlanta. Whenever I'd make it to Atlanta, I would make a special trip to see Steve and Susan. Steve did the same. He was in Orange County visiting his brother and he made a trip up to LA to see me. He and Susan had just completed a mission to Bolivia where they had built a church in a small village in the remote mountain jungles. He shared the experience. It was incredible; they were incredible. We had lunch, reminisced, swapped stories, and prayed together. In the two years of recovery, it was a high point.

Not long after that, I had another visit. Beatrice was a beautiful lady I had also met on a movie set stuck atop the Santa Monica Pier Ferris Wheel in the movie *Invisible Child* – for hours. Like Steve, Beatrice had given up on acting and moved to Modesto. I hadn't seen her in 10 years. She was in town with her seven-year-old daughter, Lexi to see the Jonas Brothers in concert. Before they headed home the next day, we got together for lunch in downtown LA. I had forgotten just how truly beautiful she was. Her smile lights up a room. She's one of those people that makes you happy to be around and Lexi took after her. We could have spent hours talking and catching up, but they had to get on the road before dark. But I was thankful for the time we shared.

The visits from Steve and Bea recharged me and my faith that had been slowly slipping since I met Beth. Then it happened – a steep, fast, downhill slide on the roller coaster ride that I had been on for the past two years. One night in the middle of August, I came across a post on the Acoustic Neuroma Forum from Crookedsmile. Her real name was Angie; Crookedsmile was her Forum screen name. She had a right to call herself that. She had the identical facial issues that I had – only on the other side. Hers were actually worse and more devastating. She was a pretty thirty-something mother of two young boys from Arkansas who had AN surgery six months before mine. I followed her recovery on the Forum over the years and it seemed like she was having a rough time of it. I never realized just how rough until she posted a series of recovery pictures on the Forum. A picture of her early in her recovery was heartbreaking. Half her face was contorted into a snarl. As the pictures progressed, she had improved to the point where the snarl was gone and her eyes, after some surgery, were about normal. However, she, like I, didn't attempt a full smile – it just wouldn't work.

Angie had been faithful in posting updates of her recovery on the Forum. But on that night in mid-August, the news was crushing. The heading to the post read: "Answers from my facial retrainer re:synkinesis and therapy."

Here's her transcript from the Forum post:

I asked the questions that have weighed heavily on my mind this entire time but didn't ask because I didn't want to hear the answers.

Q- Is synkinesis something that eventually goes away or is it here to stay......forever?

A- It is something that you will have forever but with therapy and botox we can control it to the best of our ability. The facial nerve was damaged and while regenerated it made a few bad turns hooking up to the wrong muscles in the face. That can't be changed.

Q-So once I retrain my facial muscles this isn't a permanent fix?

A-No. It is just like fitness training. Once you stop you can lose everything you gained. You will have to always do these exercises to keep things in check.

Q-Do you think that the facial nerve can recover any after the 2 year mark?

A-I believe that anything after the 2 year mark is pushing it. I believe it is pretty much done but then you have to focus on strengthening the muscles that did get reinnervated.

I was stunned. The room started spinning around me. It couldn't be. I was going to get better again – wasn't I? I'd be able to smile again – wouldn't I? Maybe her physical therapist was wrong. I immediately forwarded the post on to my PT asking if this was indeed true. I didn't hear back from her. It wasn't until that day in her office that she casually referred to Angie's message and dropped the "never" bomb.

Normally I would have been horrified at the realization. But by now I had become numb to bad news. My soul had been sucked dry of caring. I suppose if I had been younger like Angie with a long life ahead of her,

I would have been crushed. But at 61, I had had my fun in life and only had so many years left that I would have to deal with a distorted face. So I finally had the whole truth, unless of course there is some other tidbit of doom lurking out there that I don't know about.

Here's a quick look at the prognosis chart as it had been dished out to me:

Recovery Time

	Two Months	**One Year**	**Two Years**	**Never**
Face	Nope	Nope	Nope	Yep
Balance	Nope	Nope	Nope	Yep
Hearing	N/A	N/A	N/A	Yep

If I were one of those prognosticators, I stay away from gambling casinos.

What made this news so tough to deal with was the fact that up until that moment, throughout this entire two-year story to this point, I had believed that all the physical therapy I was going through, all the home exercises I was doing, all the hope that I had to be normal again someday, was not going to happen. And the term "about normal" meant a life with a disfigured face, adding to that, little balance. Maybe I was the last to realize it, but it wasn't cool. For the rest of my life, I would never smile again.

While I don't give names of medical providers in this story, I do want to mention one thing. My Physical Therapist is a sweet woman and I am sure it pained her greatly to be the bearer of bad tidings. She's just the one that was stuck holding the confession bag. I certainly don't hold it against her.

CHAPTER SIX

Back to One

February 3, 2010

In the movie business, the term "back to one" is a direction to actors and cameras to return to their starting positions to re-shoot the scene. Today I was going back to one.

Pre-surgery memories came drifting back as I pulled up to the studio gate at the entrance to the parking garage. It was here at The Lot, a production studio in Hollywood proper, that three years earlier I was Jack Nicholson's stand-in on the movie, *The Bucket List*. I didn't know it at the time that I had a tumor brewing in my brain that was playing havoc with my ability to work as a stand-in. Now I was back with a problem face, little balance, and a lack of hearing to take another stab at life in front of the cameras. I could be facing a disaster in the making.

Not long after I got the "never" news, I realized that what I was waiting to happen just wasn't going to happen and that I needed to get on with my new life as best I could. The first thing I needed to take care of was driving and to get serious about going back to work. The last time I had driven was the day before my surgery. I had grown weary of

Public Transportation buses, shuttles, and trains and having my knees painfully jammed into the seat in front of me while malodorous drunks in the seat next to me slurred rambling philosophical discussions in my deaf ear. Although I had become a proficient rider, I wanted to kick the bus-train-shuttle blues.

I hadn't attempted driving because as a passenger I would see things like cars coming toward me that were actually going the other way. This is not a good thing if you're behind the wheel of a 2000 pound machine. Forum members had different versions of what driving was like. Those with serious balance issues tended to agree that it was a bit of a challenge. Only later did they mention the impossibility of night driving.

The first thing I needed to start driving again was a car. I had rid myself of my car sometime ago when I felt it would be quite awhile before I could drive again – and it was difficult making payments to a credit company that wouldn't work with me and paying auto insurance on a car that was just sitting gathering dirt. As it happened, a co-worker of Britannia's was selling a newly rebuilt classic 1986 Pontiac Fiero GT. I had owned a Fiero in the 80's and loved it until a drunk driver plowed into it at an intersection and it never drove the same. Since I was going through my third or fourth mid-life crisis, it sounded like a good idea and a week later I bought the car. A year later it has proven to be a good idea and an excellent investment.

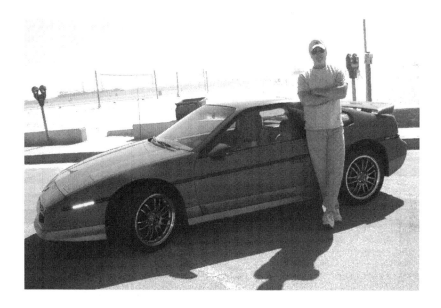

The Car

I picked up the car on a Sunday in late September. With Britannia following me in contact by cell, I ventured out onto a freeway, something I would never have given a thought to in years past. This was different. Two years earlier, my brain had been trifled with and I was still dealing with the aftermath. While I easily handled the mechanics of driving, my brain was trying to cope with its new surroundings. I can only describe it as playing a video game – involved but not totally in control. I stayed in the slow lane with both hands firmly gripping the wheel. Once Britannia was certain that I could handle it, she peeled off and headed home leaving me careening through space willy-nilly at death-defying speeds upwards of 50 miles per hour.

My first driving adventure was to head south to Lake Forest in southern Orange County to meet Samantha, my best friend from my advertising days in Atlanta. I hadn't seen her since 2002 when we had just finished running the 4th of July Peachtree Road Race together. Since that time she had gotten married and had recently had her first baby. She was in town interviewing for a marketing position that was to be based in the Southeast.

I gingerly crawled my way in the very slow lane along the 15 miles on I-5 under a brilliant Orange County sky to her hotel. I got there just as her shuttle pulled up. It was just as incredible as seeing Steve and Beatrice a month earlier. I realized that in spite of the things that had gone wrong there were a lot of things that had gone right – especially having the chance to get together with these three amazing friends.

As I drove her to dinner, she became the first passenger in my car – a daring soul – probably a bit more than she realized. We passed the hours away reliving the old; sharing the new. Suddenly I realized it was getting dark. I had a 40-mile drive ahead and I didn't want to risk driving in the dark the first time out. I took Sam back to her hotel and headed home. The sun was fading fast. I didn't make it. About halfway home, the night came down.

Driving up I-5 to Los Angeles is challenge enough. Now it was a nightmare. I found myself on a carnival ride spinning wildly through the middle of a Pink Floyd light show. My brain that had found a comfort zone for the past two years went into shock. I expected to hear from deep in my cranial recesses the iconic, "I'm sorry, Dave. I'm afraid I can't do that."

Most of the drive was a straight shot passing through the southern LA towns from Buena Park to East LA. Then what had been maddening chaos transformed itself into utter catastrophe as I veered off onto the Hollywood Freeway. Suddenly I was thrown into a frantic NASCAR world of twists and turns and bumper-to-bumper traffic racing up the freeway through downtown Los Angeles. I gripped the wheel tightly, broke into a cold sweat and tightened my seatbelt anticipating the 20 car pileup that I was doomed to participate in.

Fifteen minutes of mayhem later, I was home, parked on a silent, darkened street. I turned off the engine, sat quietly for a while, and said a prayer of thanks to God. I checked back with the balance issue folks on the Forum to see if they had similar driving experiences. They all said they never drove at night if they didn't have to. Now they tell me.

At about the same time as the auto misadventure, Los Angeles had gone through a heat spell touching off wild fires that were raging in the mountains raining down ash and smoke on Los Angeles. One morning during the spell, I woke to find my hearing in my "good ear" to be all but gone. Even with a hearing aid I couldn't understand people and had to rely totally on reading lips. I also noticed that my balance was wildly off kilter. I was getting worse and there seemed to be no reason for it. I waited a week to see if my hearing improved. It didn't. I made an appointment with my internist.

"Allergies," he said. The smoke and the ash and the heat had carried something that I was allergic to. Inner ear congestion was blocking my hearing and throwing off my balance. *Naw*, I thought. *Can't be that easy.* He prescribed a bunch of stuff. I still doubted him. I began taking the medicine. Nothing happened. I doubted him even more. Then one day I could hear as well as I normally do. It only lasted an hour but I realized he was right, I hadn't lost my hearing. Over time I've come to realize that during most of the year, my off-kilter balance is manageable. But once I run into the heat spells of August and September, all balance hell breaks loose

I had more good news that fall, I had my five-year lower gastro thing. After the procedure, my gastro doc pronounced me perfect. That was the first time in 20 years there hadn't been at least one issue. Now before I go on, I want to take this opportunity to make a Public Service Announcement. Yes, the prep is annoying but the procedure is a breeze and you spend the rest of the day in a dreamy catatonic state. If you're over 50, have a colonoscopy every five years. It doesn't hurt and it could save your life.

I had more good news. I had my first physical since I had my pre-surgery physical two years earlier. I passed with flying colors. All the good stuff was high and all the bad stuff was low. The only health issues I had at this point in my life were the result of the surgery.

That fall was a culmination of all the things I had jumped into over the past two years. Physical Therapy visits, Botox shots, meeting with AN patients at St Vincent's, visits to the gym, grilling out at Cindy's, dinners at James and Tracie's, Runyon Canyon hikes, a breakfast with my casting agent, Jessica, and running on Saturday mornings with Britannia on the Wilson High School track in Long Beach. Those runs with her paid off. On Thanksgiving morning, she and I ran the Turkey Trot along the beach in Belmont Shore. It was a full-circle event. We had last run it two years earlier a week before my surgery. But where I had to coax Britannia along the first time, she now had to coax me along. We did it. Maybe not as pretty as times earlier, but we ran the three miles.

Then came the great news. Britannia was promoted and given her own mall leasing program. But that wasn't the only good news. Her new mall was in Westwood, back in Los Angeles. On January 2, I drove a U-Haul truck down to Long Beach, packed her up, and moved her into a place a few short miles from me. I hadn't driven a U-Haul since long before my surgery. A challenge would be putting it mildly. Another milestone. But the biggest test was yet to come.

On a bright, chilly morning on February 3rd, over two years after I had last set foot in a movie studio, I headed out on a short three mile drive through Hancock Park to the streets of Hollywood to a film studio called The Lot. In the golden days of Hollywood, the studio was initially called the Pickford-Fairbanks Studio, then Warner Brothers Hollywood, and today just The Lot. A bunch of famous movies were shot there including *The Thief of Baghdad, Some Like It Hot, West Side Story, Basic Instinct, The Green Mile,* and *The Bucket List* – which I worked on.

The Lot is a small studio by Hollywood standards. Compared to the massive studios like Paramount, Warner Brothers and Sony, it's a cozy place occupying less than a single Hollywood block with just a handful of stages.

I pulled into the four-story parking structure where nearly three years earlier we filmed the pyramid scene on *The Bucket List* on the roof of the garage on a fabricated pyramid made of heavy-duty Styrofoam. No, it wasn't shot in Egypt. The scenery behind Jack and Morgan was actually West LA and Century City.

I made the very short walk to the stage where *The Social Network* was being shot and checked in with a production assistant. Today I was doing "background" (more commonly known as working as an Extra). I could no longer do stand-in work because of my hearing loss. I could no longer do Principal work because I couldn't smile. So today I was background playing a businessman in a blue or grey suit. That's about as descriptive as it gets when you are for the most part, a blur.

The stage we would be working on was the stage where the Buddhist Temple scene in Nepal was shot on the *Bucket List*. (No, we weren't in Nepal. And we weren't looking out at a snowstorm shrouded Himalayan mountain range. We were staring at a massive green screen that covered the entire stage wall). As I stepped on the stage, I paused for a moment. I was struck with an odd sensation. When I last took that step, it was another day, another job, and I had no inkling of what lay ahead several months later. Three years later, my world had changed. I wasn't the same person walking onto that stage.

I was early so I headed over to the catering truck on the other side of the lot. One of the perks in the movie business is catered meals. You can get most any breakfast you can dream up. I was nervous. I had toast. On the walk to catering, I could tell my balance was out of whack – not the stumbling around kind but the kind that I had to concentrate on to walk a straight line.

I ran the Background gamut. I went to the wardrobe trailer and checked with them. Generally, background actors supply their own wardrobe unless the production is a period piece. They liked the suit I was wearing – a blue, pin-striped Hart Schaffner and Marx with a grey shirt and a burgundy tie. But they didn't like my socks. They had a gold stripe around the toe. Seriously, people – my socks??? The camera was going to see my socks??? My friends in this business can probably guess what I was dealing with. Not that any of it matters much when you're a blur wearing something blue.

That task finished, I crossed the driveway to the hair and make-up trailer. The makeup artist seemed a little puzzled by the paralyzed corner of my mouth and my unintended arch of my eyebrow. Not that she said anything but I could sense her hesitation as she applied make-up unsure of how to make me look normal. If she could pull that off, I'd be forever indebted to her. She did her best.

Now that I was all approved for the camera, I headed back to the stage. There were just two of us in the background that day – me and a low-keyed guy named Brad. We started rehearsal almost immediately. Our action – it's the end of the work day and Brad and I were leaving the building outside a conference room where Rashida Jones was meeting with Jesse Eisenberg. It's the last scene in the movie. (If you look closely, when Rashida enters the conference room, a blue blur passes the conference room window behind Jesse. That's me).

That started it – a day of non-stop crossing through the hallway and exiting the building. The office was actually constructed on a wood platform in the middle of a darkened sound stage. Once we walked out the exit door, we immediately had to make our way down a wobbly wooden stairway in the dark – a balance ordeal to say the least.

David Fincher is an excellent director and very diligent. Very diligent. That scene was going to be perfect even if it took a thousand takes (which seemed like it did). And like a pro, Rashida, with a bunch of dialog, delivered take after take. I, on the other hand, wasn't faring well. My balance was bad. I did my best not to stagger through the lobby. I told Brad what I was dealing with and he helped out. Finally, after six tedious hours, we broke for lunch.

That day was the final day of Principal photography. What that means is that while there would be more work like inserts and technical shots, none of the Principal actors would be working and a lot of the crew wouldn't be needed. So on their last day of work, they were treated (I was included) to a special lunch; Steak Diane and Lobster Tail. On my first day back, I lucked out with a catering coup – a big deal in the background business since most of us live off thrown together meals when we get home from work and lobster doesn't appear in that mishmash.

After the lunch break, we headed back to the stage for more of the same thing – six hours of the same non-stop walking thing. We finally wrapped after a 12 hour day at 8:00 at night. I was exhausted but I did it. My first day back in the business after over two years wasn't the same, but then again it wasn't the disaster that it could have been.

CHAPTER SEVEN

Swimming with Dolphins

June 15, 2010

We were snorkeling about 50 yards off shore in Puuhanna Bay exploring the reefs and checking out a rainbow of tropical fish that were darting aimlessly through ocean floor caverns when Britannia motioned to me. She pointed to the north end of the crystal blue bay much farther out where a group of swimmers was headed. "Dolphins," she shouted over the rolling waves.

Several weeks after my first job in the acting business, I was at it again. This time I was working on the streets of downtown LA on a TV promo for the show *Leverage*. The call time was early at 6:00. If anyone believes the Hollywood production life is all glamour, they are sadly mistaken. Most days are early and long. This day was no exception. I had to drive in the dark, something that was very disorienting. I dreaded it. Fortunately I live just five miles from downtown and the streets were all well-lighted. I followed the yellow production signs to a garage on the edge of the city. I parked on the floor reserved for us and made my way down to the base camp at the garage entrance.

Hell in the Head

Base camp in the film production business is the prep area. Generally situated on a large parking lot, it is home to the star's trailers, wardrobe and hair and make-up trailers, changing rooms, and catering. Most people gravitate to the catering truck. By the time I showed up, there was already a group gathered there. They were faceless voices in the dark. Then as the dawn threw a golden glow across the group, I suddenly recognized a lot of old commercial acting buddies that I hadn't seen in over two years. We were all older, but not much else had changed. Except for Ken.

Ken was a charming Black man, a bit older than I am, who is a very well-recognized actor especially for his print advertising work. Over the years we had developed an old-guy camaraderie. During the time I had been out of work dealing with my surgery aftermath demons, Ken had been dealing with his own health issues – a stroke. He had been in the Army Honor Guard in his youth – tall and ram-rod straight. Now he was stooped with an uncertain walk. We made a pair, two old guys, a bit out of whack looking out for each other as we walked back and forth on a city street while Timothy Hutton and gang "exploded" an armored car across the street from us.

It was a long day and it got even longer. The director kept me to do another scene after the others were wrapped. For another hour, I sauntered down the street in front of the camera twirling a gold pocket watch. I have no idea to this day why. At 8:00 at night, I was finally wrapped ending another long day.

Things got quite for awhile. I slipped back into the routine of gym, running, hiking, and turning 62. Then in April, I went back to work on the movie, *Gulliver's Travels,* playing a Lilliputian butler running one way to put out a fire, then suddenly running the other way from a giant Gulliver. The running part was a challenge since my balance wasn't up to par and I was wearing Victorian era dress shoes that had a bit more of a heel than I was used to.

We shot the scene at Twentieth Century Fox Studios in Century City on the old *Chicago Hope* stage. It brought back memories. Thirteen years earlier, that stage had been the first sound stage I worked on in the television business. I did a scene in a bar where Mark Harmon's character fell off the wagon with his gambling addiction. I haven't seen *Gulliver's Travels* yet to know if that scene made the movie. If it did, I'm sure that it lasted about a second.

When I decided to go back to work, I had thought that three or four days of work per month would be the norm; actually all I could deal with. Wrong. May was as dead as March. With the exception of an audition on *Mad Men* (which I blew), the month was another month of tedium.

There was a learning experience that month. I had qualified for Medicare in March. I was now wandering aimlessly through the confusing medical Medicare maze. Someday I'll probably figure it out. Most things post-surgery have become a bit puzzling. Perhaps it has something to do with my brain being messed with.

June was Hawaii. A year earlier, my brother, Rick transferred from the mainland to Hawaii to take a job as head of Human Resources for the Kona Brewing Company. He and his wife, Nancy, their dog, Angel and four cats settled in Kona on the Big Island. Britannia and I planned a visit for his 60th birthday. So on a cool June Gloom LA morning, Britannia and I headed for the tropical sun of Hawaii. I hadn't been there in 15 years and even that visit was on business (which really isn't like being in Hawaii, it's just someplace else on business). Britannia had never been there.

I was concerned about the flight since it was first I had taken post-surgery. I had heard stories about how difficult it was to navigate the aisles of an airplane with wonkyhead (me, not the airplane). Years earlier as a regional marketing director, I spent most of 20 years in the air racking up a million miles on Delta and close to that on American. Flying was second nature. Walking an aisle on a bumpy plane was no issue. That was then and this was now. A bump and a misstep could easily send me sprawling into a row of seats – something that wouldn't particularly endear me to those whose laps I landed in. I managed to avoid any aisle walking. Stir-crazy seemed to be the only issue after the inaugural Screwdriver wore off. Three crossword puzzles could not hold the attention of my scattered brain.

We had a layover in Oahu. Hawaii was just as I remembered it – a gentle sun-drenched beauty. A few hours later we were landing at the Kona airport on the Big Island of Hawaii so named because it's the big island of the state. It's actually the island of Hawaii but that's too confusing. The island is still under construction. Unlike the other Hawaiian islands, the Big Island is home to an active volcano as well as several other recent ones – something about angry surf gods – it's all sort of confusing. As we could see on landing, much of the land resembles the moon surface covered with charcoal-gray lava flows that reach down like fingers through patches of green from the mountains to the ocean edge – quite a contrast from the tropical paradise of the other islands.

David Douglas Shannon

The Kona airport is the size of a 7-Eleven. Several steps from the plane, we were greeted with leis from Rick and Nancy. Other than seeing them for a few hours as they passed through LA on their way to Hawaii, I really hadn't spent any time with them since well before the surgery. We were a very close family and it was great being together again.

The town of Kona is an assortment of industrial parks, a "big box" retail complex, a tourist village, hotels, bars, restaurants, more bars, and homes running up the side of the mountain above it all. Rick and Nancy's home was halfway up the hillside with an expansive back deck overlooking a tropical backyard, the town below, and on to the gleaming Pacific. As we sat in silence that evening watching the sun slip below the horizon, I was struck with an odd reality. In the nearly three years since I had discovered I had a tumor, that moment was the first time I felt relaxed and at peace. I had been on a rat wheel of my own making and hadn't realized it.

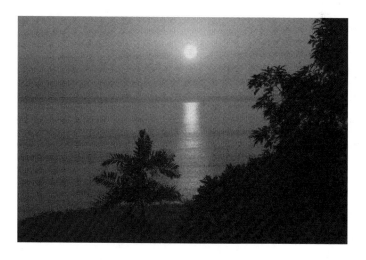

Sunset in Kona, Hawaii

The next two weeks were blissfully carefree. The only dark moment came when my hearing aid broke. A day later I had it repaired by the only audiologist in Kona. With a Kona population of 10 or 15,000, I was a bit surprised to find one there. She was a blessing.

The upsides of the stay were many. Early on I rediscovered the joy of swimming. Since the time I was young, I had always loved swimming. There was something mystical about it. But since my surgery, I feared it, probably because of the balance issues that created disorientation. On the second day we were there, Nancy took Britannia and me to a local Kona beach. I don't remember the name of it. Like all Hawaii beaches, it started with a "K" and end with an "A" with a bunch of "aumanuanama"'s in between. When I took my first dive into the water, I was ecstatic – not only because I could swim, but because I was freed from my land balance problems. It was liberating, it was thrilling, and it was the greatest I had felt physically in the past three years.

The next day the four of us traveled farther south to Puuhonua Honounau Beach, an area known for its reefs and tropical fish – ideal for snorkeling. It lay at the foot of an old lava flow which made crossing the gray craggy rock to the water a bit tough and getting off it and into the water a real ordeal. But once in the water wearing snorkel gear, I was in paradise. We spent the next hour exploring the reefs and the exotic multi-colored sea life. Then Britannia spotted a crowd of swimmers heading farther out. Suddenly she saw why they were going out as a dolphin flipped into the air. We swam out to join them. There were about 20 or 30 of us out there as the dolphins swam around and in between us. It's not permitted to interact with them but it was nevertheless just a thrill to swim around them – we knew they were friends. As simple as it may sound, that was the highpoint of the past three years.

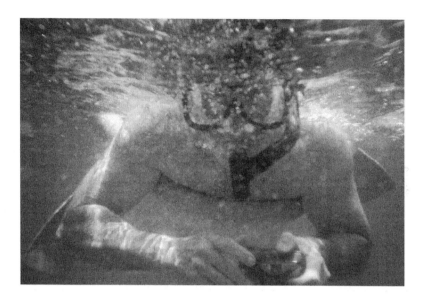

Snorkeling

There was another of those simply great moments a few days later when we drove down to the southernmost tip of the Big Island to visit the Kilauea Volcano (the active one). We entered the Hawaii Volcanoes National Park and drove along a winding two lane road through a wooded landscape ending up at a Welcome Center where we felt welcomed. From there we drove farther up the hill to the Kilauea Caldera in which the Halemaumau Crater sits. There is a museum next to the Caldera. While we were there the crater began to spew white smoke (which I am quite sure was poisonous) billowing into the air. This of course was all strange to me. I'm no scientist but I do know that volcanoes blow up. I've flown over Mt. St Helens and saw how nasty they can be. So why would anyone put a welcome center and a museum on top of an active volcano and invite people there to their doom? Since no one could answer that question in a way a simple guy like me could understand, I just had to assume that I was spending my last day on Earth. As it was, I guess it was my lucky day since I got off that volcano without being blown up into the universe.

Before we left, my brother and I tossed a football around. This was one of those "did you ever imagine that you would someday be playing football on top of an active volcano" moments.

I had another one of those moments an hour later at the bottom of the volcano by the edge of the ocean as we walked across a lava flow that had been in an active area between 2004 and 2007. I was actually walking on land that was three years old. I'm not impressed with the stuff that most people are. I like the simple things. Swimming with dolphins and walking across newly formed land were just those simple things. There would be one other event later that year that would match that simple joy.

I spent the next two weeks with Rick, Nancy and Britannia traveling to different beaches, eating at the Kona Brewing Pub (voted best pizza on the island), and hiding out from reality. It was an amazing time and a much needed break. But like all happy and wonderful things, it came to an end and I returned home tanned and rested, resigned to resuming my post-AN life.

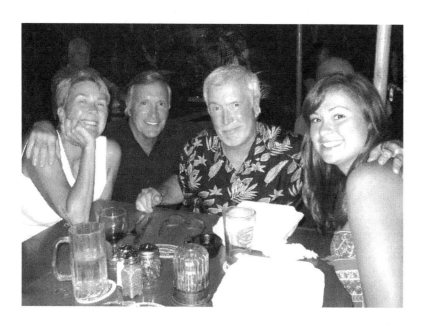

Nancy, Rick, me and Britannia at the Kona Brewing Company Pub

CHAPTER EIGHT

Crookedsmile

November 4, 2010

As much as I want to capture the moment, I couldn't do it writing justice. She and I shared a bond that no one in our lives could understand. We had supported each other through the dark times. When there was no one who knew what was in our hearts, we knew. When I finally saw her pictures on the Forum of a beautiful woman who had gone through the disfigurement of her face, I cried. When she lost her baby to a miscarriage, I cried. When she told me our facial mess was permanent, she cried. When we finally met we both cried...and laughed.

June and July are hiatus months for the film business. Generally the only projects being shot are commercials and low budget Indies when stage and equipment rental is less expensive. With the little work I had done until that point during the active filming months, I settled into a plan of writing and sorting out stuff like Medicare and other recovery issues. So it came as a surprise when I call the call several days after my return from Hawaii that I was booked on the movie *Atlas Shrugged*. The first thing that struck as being odd was that *Atlas Shrugged* was actually being made into a movie. The book by Ayn Rand weighed 30 pounds and took me two years to read – and that was the Cliff Notes version. By the time you finish the book, you have to go back and read the beginning to remember how it started. How anyone could condense that thing into a two hour or so movie was beyond me.

As I showed up for work the next morning, I discovered that the effort was going to be even more challenging. The shooting schedule was 24 days. Most movies take months to shoot. And the budget for the movie was only $5 million. That's nearly unheard of. I knew right away there were no stars in the movie. A five million salary alone would hardly be enough to attract them. Apparently, after 20 years of having the rights to make the movie, the rights were about to expire and the producer had to put something together or lose them. (At least that was what I understood. I have since heard other versions).

Taking that and the schedule and the budget into account, I knew what to expect before setting foot on the set – chaos. Fourteen hours of chaos to be exact. It came from inexperience. The crew, the production team, the directors, the actors were all trying to figure things out on the fly since they hadn't had the time to prepare. The only one who seemed to have the slightest clue was the caterer since this was just another movie for them. For background actors like me, it was even more confusing since we were tossed into the jumble for just a day.

After 12 hours of misdirection and walking back and forth in front of the camera to have the scene suddenly changed, my balance had become horrendous. For the last two hours, I was a business executive walking through the office lobby on my way home. I looked more like a business executive stumbling out of an office party attempting to appear normal – unsuccessfully. Mercifully, it came to an end at 1:00 in the morning after 14 hours of crazy.

Then, a few days later, I got a call that I would be playing a taxi driver on *Mad Men*. Cold sweat time. Would I have to drive? And if I had to drive, would I have any of the principal actors as passengers? And should I mention to anyone that my head was all messed up and who knows, I just might veer off the side of a cliff? Nothing like being a neurotic mess for a few days.

The day came and I had a late afternoon call time at LA Center Studios. The studio sits just on the edge of downtown LA about a mile from St Vincent's Hospital. It's one of the newer studios in town that developed from the adjoining, formerly deserted, Unocal office building that had been occasionally leased out for filming. In past years I worked there on movies such as *Nurse Betty, The Klumps, Pirates of Silicon Valley*, and a bunch of other ones that get jumbled together in mind-numbing sameness. Today the studio is the home of *Mad Men* and *Law and Order LA*.

In the Background world waiting is the norm. This was no exception. I waited alone for five brain-killing hours. Over the years I've learned to keep my mind alive by doing crossword puzzles and guessing what the mystery food was on the Craft Service table without the courage to actually eat it.

Finally at midnight, they were ready to shoot the taxi scene I was in. The company made a move to a stage – which meant that I fortunately would not have to drive. The taxi was mounted on rollers to give the impression of movement while stage lights flashed by as if they were headlights from passing cars. Since the scene was set at night, the stage was largely dark. I would just have to give the impression of driving – which was also fortunate because I think Jon Hamm and a lady companion were in the back seat (I didn't turn around to check). I don't think the producer would have been too thrilled if I had gone careening down the street with two of the stars' lives in jeopardy.

But one concern was replaced with another. Since the day that I had gone back to work, I had been dreading the moment when my crooked face would actually be on camera. The camera was placed just at the end of the hood of the taxi. There was no escaping it. While the scene was being set up, an assistant director kept coming over to me as I sat behind the wheel in the taxi and told me to relax. I was relaxed. I enjoy being on camera. But I don't think she was interested in hearing about how brain tumor surgery caused Synkinesis and how because my nerves rewired wrong, my face looks tense. I did what I could do appear relaxed by casually leaning on the door. It looked just like some guy with a tense face trying to look relaxed.

We began to shoot. After each cut, the director seemed to be getting more irritated. Finally after four or five takes, he called the camera operator over. After a short discussion, an AD told me to move over against the door and the camera team moved the camera so at least my face would be out of frame.

I guess my face wasn't ready for primetime or maybe primetime wasn't ready for my face. Either way, I didn't pull it off. It was a gut punch. That was the reality that I feared. At that moment I finally realized that my old life was genuinely gone. Until that point I had been saying the words but not really accepting it. I was wrapped right after that scene. I left the studio alone in the dark and drove home passing St Vincent's

Hospital on the way – the place where the ugly started.

A few weeks later in mid-July, it happened again. I was playing a father at an intimate dinner around a coffee table on the show *Enlightened* – just four of us. My son-in-law was telling us a joke. We were to laugh. The best I could manage was a lop-sided grin. But unlike the previous experience, the director didn't seem to mind and the scene came off well. It wasn't the same though. In the past, I would have put all of me into that scene – and I would have loved doing it.

Then the work stopped. I wasn't being cast. It's true that a lot of film production had moved from the overly expensive confines of California to more film-friendly states and Canada. It's also true that work for Screen Actors Guild actors had greatly been reduced with TV contracts being undercut by sister union AFTRA. But nothing. Although in reality I knew it wouldn't happen, I started to conjure up the notion that word had spread among casting directors that there was this guy out there with a messed up face and that if you didn't want to wreck a scene, don't cast him. As crazy as that may sound, the thought did go through my head.

Actually no work was a fortunate thing. My balance took a turn for the worse in August. I suppose it was seasonal allergies that were doing the damage. I live on the top floor of a five-story building and on days when the elevator isn't working because some thoughtless person left the elevator door opened (it happens a lot), I was for the most part trapped. With an out-of-whack balance system, I really didn't feel like navigating the steps. In reality, with an arthritic knee, I wasn't supposed to be using the steps anyway. (Note to self: Move). August was ugly. I wasn't working. I was having trouble with a medical billing department.

I was turning into a vegetable. I needed to break the routine.

Then I got an invitation from an old buddy from my corporate days who had a house in Summerlin overlooking the Las Vegas Strip – the perfect place to get away for a week of sunning, swimming and writing. I chanced my first flight alone – not particularly a big undertaking in that it was only an hour flight and the Bob Hope Burbank Airport terminal was small enough that it was easy to navigate and I guessed well at the PA announcements. The Las Vegas Airport on the other hand, with the constant clatter of slot machines and its sprawling terminal, wasn't quite as easy. With trusty cane in hand, I managed navigating through the circus that was Las Vegas.

The week was just as I had planned. The weather was perfect in the 90's which warmed the pool during the day for swimming. Without any other distractions, I went on a writing tear. I wrote most of this story sitting out in the sun by the pool that week.

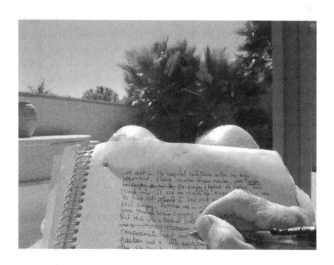

Writing poolside

I returned home to a bit of a void and a heat wave with a record high for Los Angeles of 113 degrees. Do you realize how hot 113 degrees actually is?! – especially for a place where the average annual temperature is 72 degrees and a lot of places aren't air-conditioned because of it. That was crazy. I don't think I moved an inch that day for fear of having a heat stroke.

I filled the void with visits to the gym in Hollywood and running on Saturdays with Britannia in a tree-shaded park in Beverly Hills. Then, with the encouragement of photographer friend, Michael, I took a chance. All my pre-surgery acting publicity shots showed a toothy-smile me. It would have been deceptive to continue using those shots since I could no longer duplicate that look. Michael offered to do updated shots of me with a lop-sided grin. So on a hazy afternoon in late October we did a shoot. I had done a lot of commercial print work pre-surgery and was comfortable with a camera lens. But this would be a challenge – I was missing a big part of my on-camera arsenal – my smile. We went through a bunch of looks – formal, detective, country club, military vet. Michael pulled it off – a series of normal-as-I-could-look shots that I'm now using as headshots.

David Douglas Shannon

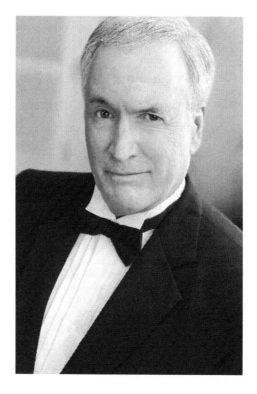

October 2010
Photography by Michael Kurtz

I also spent the downtime researching the technical parts of this book. It was during this research that I discovered some enlightening and disturbing facts.

I generally believe what people in the medical profession tell me. They know more about their subject than I do and since they tend to write in technical speak, I usually don't read much and take them at their word. For me a picture book would be nice. What I wasn't thinking is that they want your business and as a result they seem to sugarcoat, downplay, and minimize the potential post-surgery downsides all while putting the pre-surgery fear of God in you.

Here's the pre-surgery talk: *You have to have that tumor thing out, there's not much time left, you could be walking down the someday and that ticking time-bomb in your head goes WHAMMO and you're history. Oh, and by the way, there could be some post-surgery inconveniences, but don't worry, that hardly ever happens.* That of course is a slight exaggeration, but that is how I interpreted those pre-surgery discussions – so much so that as I wrote earlier, my only real concerns were how much insurance was going to cover, would I be able to return to work at the end of the Writer's Strike, and how could I go a month without blowing my nose? The rest of it would work out just the way the medical people told me. Sure it would.

The first bit of misunderstanding had to do with balance and the creation of my wonkyhead. What I understood was this; the balance nerve on the AN side will be removed during surgery but the balance nerve on the opposite side will compensate for it. Do balance exercises after you leave the hospital and everything will be fine. What I didn't hear was this; you have to seriously challenge your brain – like spend the first few weeks of walking the aisles of a Target – an un-nerving task to this day.

According to the "Improving Your Balance" brochure from the Acoustic Neuroma Association, the brain is lazy (my words, not theirs specifically). To quote the brochure specifically, here's what it actually says:

"In essence, the brain will correct the balance system only as much as it must. As long as the strategy the brain has adopted works reasonably well, it will stick with that system. For the most part, people can function reasonably well with a visual system as a priority sense for balance. It is bothersome to feel a bit unsteady or dizzy when going downstairs, walking in a crowded shopping mall or walking down a grocery store aisle where many colored boxes create the visual image of movement (no kidding), but typically these activities are not preformed enough for the brain to correct the problem."

So what this means, of the three elements of the balance system, if the brain can slide by just using the vision system and proprioceptive system (sensors in the legs and spine), it's going to by-pass redevelopment of the inner-ear system. Little did I know it at the time, but that's what I was doing during my hospital hallway walks. They were effortless for me to the surprise of everyone, including the physical therapist – my brain had already started learning the easy way out. Couple that with the fact that I had few opportunities to get out and walk in the sensory over-loaded world outside during my first two months of recovery, my balance system was doomed as it turned into a wonky-headed mess. My brain just never felt the need for the full balance system. Sure, I did the balance exercises I was given when I left the hospital, but they weren't enough. This unfortunately is something I learned three years after-the-fact. I sincerely hope it's not too late for a mid-course correction. I suppose if I had fully understood the technical aspects of the Brainport system, I might have grasped the lazy brain thing and why it needed to be trained with electronic stimulus that it understood.

Take my advice, if you are planning AN surgery, once you leave the hospital head straight for a Six Flags for a few weeks of non-stop rollercoaster and thrill-ride riding – that should send your brain a message. (Just kidding about that – that may be a tad too much. But do challenge your brain).

Other byproducts of a disturbed balance system are emotional and disorientation factors, especially when one is standing. The brain is so busy dealing with balance issues that it doesn't have the time for cognitive thought. This leads to frequent loss for words, frustration in normal conversation, inhibition, insecurity, and visual disorientation when driving, especially at night. I went from being a very fit athletic-type to a cautious old man with the wave of the whimsical AN wand.

I was recently watching an episode of NCIS where I was playing a Joint Chiefs of Staff Admiral boldly hurrying down a long set of steps behind Mark Harmon and team. I had to laugh. Today I would be over to the side of the steps holding the handrail for dear life.

For years I thought it was my brain's reaction to a five-hour surgery under anesthesia. I now understand how my vestibular system affects my thought process and why I shy away from social functions and interaction with strangers. Being deaf in one ear is tough enough. Being mostly deaf in the other is worse. An out of whack vestibular system makes it basically impossible. My brain is being overworked with basic things like maintaining balance and trying to process words spoken by others.

I bypassed my college's anniversary reunion not long ago in September. It would have been a great opportunity to get together with college friends that I hadn't seen in over 30 years. Trying to navigate airports and flight connections and car rentals would have been chaotic and tough enough. But participating in social settings with people who aren't used to the "new" me would have been a nightmare. In two days I will be driving to Las Vegas. That will be the farthest I've driven by over two hundred miles since long before my surgery. I'm hoping my brain rises to the cause.

Another little tidbit of information I came across in my research had to do with hearing aids. At one point during the recovery process over the last three years, I met with an audiologist at the clinic. She wasn't particularly forthcoming in advice about my hearing and basically referred me back to my original audiologist. But she did give me a pamphlet on hearing impairment. My hearing loss is sensorinural, meaning nerve-type loss. For this reason I can hear with the assistance of a hearing aid in my "good ear" but I can't always understand what I hear. I had believed it was the fault of my hearing aid which is the top-of-the-line Widex. As a result I rely almost exclusively on lip-reading in a conversation and limit my television viewing to news and sports where I can either see the newscaster's lips or the action on the field that is self-explanatory. Closed captioning helps but it takes a lot of effort to process everything. I came across this in the booklet from the clinic:

"The primary objective in wearing a hearing aid is to bring about more nearly normal communications in every day life. To achieve this, good speech reading is almost always required. For maximum benefits lip-reading rehabilitation should accompany the practice training in using the hearing aid."

What? Would it have been too difficult for someone to tell me that three years ago when I first got the hearing aid?

I suppose all of this is my fault for not spending ten years in medical school and filling in the blanks on my own. All along I had believed everything that was told to me by medical professionals and that was all I needed to know. I didn't really see the need for much more self-education other than the information I was getting from the Acoustic Neuroma Association forum – folks who were for the most part in the dark as much as I was. There wasn't a manual entitled "What Happens If Things Go Wrong?" (Although there should be).

It has occurred to me that medical practitioners could be stingy on information for fear of malpractice suits. If it is, I don't follow that thinking. It seems to me that a better informed patient is better able to deal with issues as they arise. For over two years I was spoon-fed bad news. It took me three years to finally get a grip on my recovery or lack thereof. Of course on a more cynical view, recovery therapy costs big bucks and I could be nothing more than a cash cow. In either case, at 62 I probably have another 15 or 20 years to deal with it. My brain had better start getting with the program or that's going to be an awfully long bumpy ride. Even as I write this, I realize just how long the last three years have been. OK, enough of my rant. To be continued in the final chapter. Let's get back to the story.

On a warm November morning when it should have been cool, I packed the Fiero with my stuff, my drugged-up cat, Yikes and her stuff and headed out on a great adventure – a road trip to Las Vegas. The last time I made that drive was in May 2007. I didn't give it much thought then. I was driving from one place to another. This time it was different. This was the first time I would make the drive since my surgery…and it was the farthest I would drive straight by about 220 miles. Driving was still the biggest test I faced. Driving at slow speeds on city streets took all the effort I could rein in. But that wasn't all I was dealing with. My car had yet to be tested on the open road for any real distance and a breakdown in the middle of the desert would be a disaster. The car may have been a classic and it may have been rebuilt, but it was still old. And then there was Yikes. She was an older easy-going cat. Not much caused her concern save a tardy dinner. Yet I really didn't know how she would take a four or five hour drive – even a bit tranquilized.

The first part of the trip was miserable. Even at 9:00 in the morning, LA traffic is a bumper-to-bumper parking lot. Who am I kidding? The only time it isn't, is somewhere around 2:00 at night. After a half hour of snaking through town, I finally made it to I-10 – the first leg of the trip to Las Vegas.

I-10 is a massive freeway that cuts through the San Gabriel Valley passing LA's eastern towns and suburbs. To the north of the highway stand the mountains of the Angeles Forest; to the south, industrial, retail sprawl. It's the major route heading east from LA used heavily by semis hauling cargo from the port of Long Beach. The road shows its wear. My car bounced down the uneven, heavily rutted road as my brain bounced along with it. A bouncing brain is not a good thing. It makes it very difficult to concentrate on the two huge semis on either side and the tailgater behind. That lasted for 40 long miles out to San Bernardino and the switchover to I-15 heading northeast to Las Vegas. I passed the bouncing brain test. The car was on trial next.

During the summer, I had a scare on a drive to a movie set as I drove up a steep highway grade in the heat. The engine started over-heating. While it wasn't yet hot, the car faced a rugged climb into the mountains and the high desert where it would be clear sailing. After a tough 30 mile climb through the Cajon Pass and on to Hesperia, the car came through like the machine of its glory days.

I passed through Victorville, home of Roy Rodgers, Dale Evans and a stuffed Trigger and on through Barstow, the halfway point. I was getting tired and my brain was getting fuzzy but I felt like I could make it with 180 miles to go. That was until a dazed Yikes roared to life. She had been riding in the seat next to me in her cat carrier. She was supposed to be out cold. She wasn't. The trouble started with a few innocent meows and quickly escalated into a full-scale carrier breakout as I cruised down the road at 80 miles an hour. Suddenly a deranged Yikes was free to roam the small confines of a two-seater sports car. I had enough trouble focusing on driving. Now I had to be concerned about the cat.

Her first stop was the litter box that I had placed on the passenger's side floor in case of an emergency. I guess this was an emergency and the reason for the breakout. Unfortunately, being so tranqed, she couldn't really stand up. Half of what she was doing ended up in the litter, the other half in her butt fur. For a moment I felt as though she would find that the litter box to be suitably comfortable and not worth the effort to crawl back into the seat. No such luck. With a great strain, she pulled herself up and sat looking at me with a very spaced-out furry face. She's generally a typical independent cat except when she gets confused. Then she gets needy. I'm guessing that the combination of the drugs and peeing at 80 miles an hour confused her a bit. With over a hundred miles to go, she crawled over the console and plopped her wet, litter-caked butt down on my lap, dazed, pawing at the steering wheel and hinting at a lunge for the brake pedal to stop the madness. Pre-surgery it would have been cute. Post-surgery it was just insane. I knew there would be no way to keep her in her carrier and even then, I would have to pull off the road in the middle of nowhere to get her back in.

My brain with its limited ability was now dealing with a 14-pound, wet-butt, ball of fur on my lap and a 2,000 pound machine barreling down the highway. I spent the next two hours concentrating on staying between the lines, avoiding smashing into the car in front of me, and guessing what Yikes was up to next. At 1:30 on November 3, we safely made it to Las Vegas. With the trip over, my thoughts turned to the reason I had made the journey and put myself through all the weirdness.

She and I had shared our lives and our trials over the past two years. We shared a bond – a very rare bond. We were the other half of our smiles – half of my smile being in Little Rock; half of hers in Los Angeles. We became friends. We knew each other's lives, disappointments, frustrations, hopes and fears. We knew the desperation of what we were left to deal with.

In the late morning, the lobby of Planet Hollywood is a quiet refuge from the clatter and roar of the dingy smoke-filled casinos. White sunlight streamed in through the soaring floor to ceiling windows creating a celestial glow. But for a few people sitting in hushed conversation, the place was empty and still.

There was some confusion. I saw a beautiful woman sitting next to another woman who could have been her mom. I had seen pictures of her before but most of them were pre-surgery and the ones post-surgery showed a contorted face, the result of Synkinesis. I was a half an hour early so I guessed it wasn't them. I sat down and called her and left a message that I was there. The two women left. Moments later I got a call.

"Where are you?" she said. The beautiful woman I had seen sitting a few moments earlier was now standing at the end of the reception area holding a cell phone to her ear. We flew across the lobby. Within seconds I was hugging the woman who had supported me through the dark times of the past three years. The one who knew what I was dealing with because she too was dealing with it. I was hugging Angie, "Crookedsmile." We had a hard time letting go of each other. There were happy tears. It was an incredible moment filled with more than I could have imagined. I met her mom, a wonderful lady who had cared for my friend through the tough times.

The three of us spent an incredible afternoon chatting over a glass of wine in a darkened, deserted lounge at Caesars Palace getting to know each other and share our lives. We compared faces which may have seemed odd but neither one of us had met another with Synkinesis. This was something new. We could see the face muscles acting up, the arched eyebrow, and the tense cheek. I was looking at myself in Angie's face – of course she was much prettier. We laughed at the irony that she had had her surgery in the Pittsburgh hospital I was born in. I learned more about her agonizing early months of recovery – something that she had never really shared before. I was talking to a very brave woman, an inspiration to me then and now.

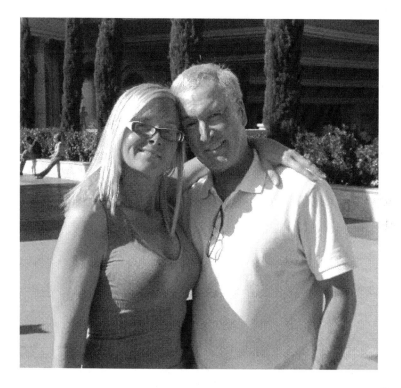

Two half smiles making one

Unfortunately our time had to come to an end. I had to get on the road before dark. We said goodbye to each other in the middle of a shopping plaza in Planet Hollywood. As we hugged, I promised that I would always be there for her. If she promised me anything, I wouldn't have heard. She would have been talking in my deaf ear. But I knew what was in her heart. I think I realized that we would probably never see each other again. She was married with a family in Little Rock, a long way from Los Angeles. But God blessed us with a chance to meet. Those four beautiful hours buried all the pain and frustration and confusion of the past three years. It was sad to say goodbye but we at least had the chance. And for me that chance was the greatest moment in a very long, dark, unforgiving time.

EPILOGUE

An Advocacy

December 3, 2010

In the cold and dark of the morning when creativity flows unrehearsed, I am finishing this part of my life. A cool breeze blows in through the window. Tangerine Dream plays across the room. It's the music I listen to when I write. Haunting and mysterious. I'm up before dawn. I wanted to see the sunrise break across the Los Angeles skyline just as I did three years ago as I was being wheeled to surgery. Today is the third anniversary of my surgery. I felt like it was a good time to end this story. I could probably go on writing but it would just be more of the same so I chose to finish things with meeting Angie in Las Vegas. A fitting end.

It's been a very long three years…very long. Just reliving it through writing was exhausting. The experience would be impossible to sum up in words only to say that it was far more than I could ever imagine. I wish I could say I'm a better person for it. I'm not. If I were, I would have moved on. Those around me have long ago accepted my crooked face, my deafness, and my wacky balance. I haven't. It's something I live with every day. Whenever I try to smile, whenever I get behind the wheel of a car, whenever I'm closed out of a conversation because I can't hear, I'm reminded of it. I've become unsure and insecure in social settings and have found myself becoming a recluse comfortable in my own surroundings. I tend to keep company only with close friends and haven't really invited any one new into my life and have even distanced myself from those who couldn't accept what I was going through.

But as much as has gone wrong, even more has been good. I've been blessed with friends and family who care. I've been blessed with financial security while I sort out things. I've been blessed with the chance to meet beautiful survivors like Angie and Beth – my support and inspiration. I've learned that all AN survivors have my back. I've learned – probably a bit more than I wanted to know about the medical profession. I've learned that I've taken a lot for granted. Something as simple as a smile has become a precious memory. And very importantly, I'm not in pain. As I have discovered over the years, there are survivors who live with daily headache pain. Whatever pain I have is of my own making.

As I was writing this story, I began to wonder just why I was writing it. Was it some sort of cathartic therapy? Or was it some sort of elongated pity-me session? Then I realized its possible purpose. In the last chapter I mentioned that there was no manual for "When Things Go Wrong." Maybe this is that manual. If it hasn't already become apparent, I'm a bit disappointed with the preparation for the surgical downside provided by the medical profession. It wasn't as though they were deceptive. It was more like the downsides were something of an afterthought. Something that happened so rarely that it wasn't worth the effort to go into. But does it happen so rarely?

When I was in Hawaii getting my hearing aid fixed, I told the audiologist that I had had an Acoustic Neuroma surgery. She looked at me and made a motion to the side of her face and said, "You were lucky, you didn't get the…." Then I half smiled and she said "Oh, I'm sorry, you did." That seemed a bit unusual to me that she would reference facial paralysis as something common. So I researched this. What exactly were the downsides and the associated percentages? According to data compiled by Chicago Dizziness and Hearing affiliated with Northwestern University, here are the percentages of complications due to Acoustic Neuroma surgery:

- Stroke (rare). I know of three – Angie, Beth, and Kay.
- Injury to cerebellum, pons or temporal lobe (rare).
- Death (about 1/2 percent to 2 %, depending on the center).
- CSF leak (5-15 percent of all patients). I know of several.
- Meningitis (2-10 percent).
- Facial weakness (4 to 15 percent incidence of total paralysis). Tumor size is a large factor in this complication. I know a bunch with some sort of paralysis.
- Hearing loss risk (immediately after surgery).
  - Translabyrinthine -- 100%
  - Retrosigmoid -- 60%
  - Middle fossa - -40%. Hearing occasionally improves for the middle fossa approach (Stidham and Roberson, 2001).
- Headache (persistent in 10-34 percent, Ruckenstein et al 1996; Soumekh et al, 1996)

- Imbalance and dizziness (almost all patients who have any vestibular function prior to surgery, will have worsening of balance after surgery). This is not a complication, but a consequence.

He goes on to say this about balance:

This is simple stuff -- balance deteriorates after acoustic surgery because the surgery damages or removes remaining function in the vestibular nerve (Levo et al, 2004; Tufarelli et al, 2007). Tufarelli and associates reported that 10% of 459 patients judged their imbalance as disabling, and 73% felt that they had at least moderate oscillopsia (trouble seeing with head moving).

It has been our experience that over the long term (i.e. 2 years), balance generally returns to near normal, but persons who have other deficits such as visual disturbances (e.g. cataract), sensory loss (e.g. neuropathy), brain damage (e.g. cerebellar or brainstem damage due to the tumor or surgery), or poor adaptation (e.g. due to advanced age) may never obtain complete return of balance.

And just to round things out, a few more tidbits courtesy of the Michigan Ear Institute:

TASTE DISTURBANCE AND MOUTH DRYNESS
Taste disturbance and mouth dryness are not uncommon for a few weeks following surgery. In 5% of patients this disturbance is prolonged.

OTHER NERVE WEAKNESSES

Acoustic tumors may contact the nerves which supply the eye muscles, the face, the mouth and throat. These areas may be injured with resultant double vision, numbness of the throat, weakness of the face and tongue, weakness of the shoulder, weakness of the voice and difficulty swallowing. These problems may be permanent.

"Hmmm," Dave hmmmed to himself.

Why did I not hear of most of this stuff? I guess I was amiss in not researching prior to surgery but foolishly I just assumed that I would be told everything I needed to know. Of course if I knew the mess that was awaiting me, I'm sure I would have run the other way like a scared rabbit. By the way, sorry for bogging this narrative down with statistics, but it needed to be said.

In any case, I have to believe I'm not alone in what I knew or didn't know prior to surgery. As I have mentioned before, the Acoustic Neuroma Association forum is a valuable resource for pre-op patients... that is if they knew it existed. I didn't. I discovered it much after the fact. I got hit with a lot of stuff post-surgery. I'd suggest that anyone who is planning an AN surgery head to the Forum first to get input on firsthand experiences. The participants may not be experts but they can steer you in the right direction. Here's the link:

http://www.anausa.org/smf/

Unfortunately I don't believe those in the medical fields completely grasp the aftermath of complications and clearly define them. Their concern is the surgery and the immediate care. Based on the inquires on the Forum, it seems like I wasn't the only one in the dark following surgery. As I experienced, it seems like quite a few people were sent home from the hospital with little more than a list of prescriptions, a sheet of balance exercises, and a vague understanding of what could happen. No amount of optimism could have prepared me for what did happen and my confusion. After three years, I feel like I've received all the bad news I'm going to get – but it would have been so much easier to deal with it if I had been better prepared.

Now here's the purpose for this book (I finally figured it out). Here's what I'm advocating:

1. Clinics and medical providers who are responsible for the surgeries need to provide a broader scope of the potential surgery consequences. As I have been witness to, it has been more like a factory mentality. You have a tumor, we're taking it out on such and such date, there may be complications, here's a pamphlet (which by the way did not go into anywhere near the potential for disaster). To quote a brochure that I received prior to surgery – "there may be facial weakness." Such an understatement. Three of us, Nancy, Lanie and I meet unofficially with patients prior to surgery – usually the day before. There is an incredible amount of information they weren't aware of. This should be done in an official capacity.

2. While the hospital did provide a physical therapist to help with vestibular rehabilitation in the hospital and a sheet of balance exercises to take home, as I discovered, that wasn't sufficient. The patient needs to be provided a greater

understanding of the intricacies of the balance system. I don't know for certain, but I'm guessing that if I had known more about what the brain required to adjust, I would be much better off today. A simple "the remaining balance nerve will compensate" isn't sufficient. While I don't know this for a fact, I believe individuals have different degrees of balance. Athletes have keener and more refined systems. Everyone should not be treated the same. A base-line measurement of the vestibular system should be assessed pre-surgery and a customized post-surgery vestibular rehabilitation program should be developed on that base-line. A sheet of exercises may not be appropriate for some. I've been an athlete all my life. Up until surgery, even at 59, I was still a proficient sprinter. Now I am far from it. Had my system been analyzed pre-surgery and identified as being more highly-tuned, perhaps a program could have been developed to meet those specialized demands. There is a bothersome phrase used by post-operative patients – "new normal." I don't think that's acceptable.

3. It is true that there are only a few therapists trained in facial reanimation, but whenever possible, such a therapist should be brought in for counseling immediately whenever the facial nerve has been affected during surgery. I was sent home with "you'll be fine in a month or two." Three years later, I'm not fine. During my early recovery when half my face was entirely paralyzed, I found a list of exercises for the face on the Bells Palsy site. I did those exercises up to and including regaining nerve action in my face. I don't know this for a fact, but now I

suspect those exaggerated exercises may have been the cause of the Synkinesis. Had I known about this in advance, it may have been preventable.

4. Access to a psychologist who specializes in traumatic stress disorders should be made available. Speaking for myself, I am quite sure my anti-social tendencies aren't normal and are a by-product of post-surgery issues. I feel like if this had been headed off earlier in the process, I wouldn't be left to coping in my own dysfunctional way. I've also witnessed a variety of emotional discord in others who have been left to deal with their own demons – whether it be cynicism, relationship issues, depression or a fatalistic emotional detachment – they could have been professionally handled. I know of one young girl who was going through a divorce which she blamed on the aftermath of her AN surgery.

According to psychiatrist Dr. Elizabeth J. S. Kunkel who spoke at the ANA's National Symposium in July 2007, "17 to 55% of people with an Acoustic Neuroma experience depression...depression is a common problem with Acoustic Neuromas...complications with the seventh cranial nerve (facial nerve) result in disfigurement with some...disfigurement has social consequences in how people relate to you. It may make people isolate themselves and impair self-esteem; this seems to be particularly true for younger patients and women (and actors – that's my observation, not hers)."

This seems to a bigger issue that wasn't even addressed. And as a side-note to caregivers, while it shouldn't be necessary to walk on eggshells, just be cognizant of the fact that the one you are caring for may be going through an emotional rollercoaster that they are trying to cope with. And while they may be functioning normally on the outside, there's a turmoil within that's still looking for answers and peace.

5.   And finally, there is the "up front, what if" negotiations. When surgery is being negotiated among the medical providers and insurers and patients, post-operative care should also be negotiated so the patient knows going in to the surgery that they are covered in case they need to be. My insurer was quite good. There was only a slight misunderstanding when it came to Botox injections. But from the experiences of others, that's not always the case. The clinic or medical provider who is responsible for the surgery should take a vested interest and joint responsibility for post-operative care instead of a "wash your hands" approach to the matter. In my case, eye care was immediate and well-maintained. Protection of the cornea was after all a medical necessity. But there are a host of other issues that may need to be addressed as well and the patient shouldn't be left to fend for themselves. It's tough enough dealing with the surgery let alone the consequences.

Now of course, I don't know whether all this is possible or conceivable. But in my vision of a perfect world, it would happen. And for all I know, it may already be happening – that wasn't my experience. For most of my first year post-surgery, I felt like a ping pong ball in a spinning clothes dryer. I didn't like that and I don't think it was necessary.

Obviously, according to the percentages, most people breeze through the surgery with little to deal with on the other side. They go back to normal functioning lives. But then there are those like me that got a bit more than they bargained for.

As a follow-up to the last chapter, Yikes and I made it back safely from Las Vegas. This time she slept all the way to my relief. The car once again was a dream to drive. Angie and I wrote back and forth after returning but soon both of us got tied up in Thanksgiving and the holidays and drifted out of touch. I know when things settle down, it'll be back to normal. I spent Thanksgiving with Britannia. We continue to run together every Saturday.

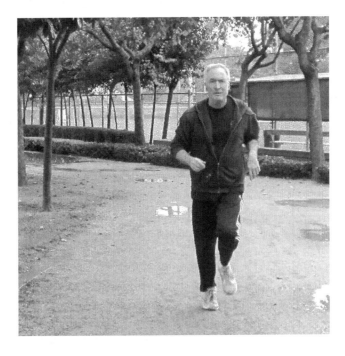

A Saturday morning run in the park.

I worked on a French movie called *The Artist* not long after returning from Las Vegas. It required a lot of walking up and down a stairway and my balance was particularly bad. Not fun, but it was work. And of course, I'm still trying to figure out Medicare and I'm running out of time. Seems like every time I get a bead on things, they up and move the target.

I've been writing this epilogue since 5:00 this morning, just about the time Britannia and I showed up at the hospital three years ago today. It's now just after 3:00 in the afternoon; I was out of surgery by now just heading out on the road of a different life. I'm still on that road. In spite of occasional nasties, it's been a journey of rich and wonderful experiences. I've met some amazing and beautiful people who share the bond of the post-AN surgery world as crazy as it is. One of them, Debbi who also has facial paralysis, left a message on Facebook today in response to my post that this was my third anniversary. She said "I never, EVER thought that I would be celebrating brain surgery anniversaries." She said it best. Brain tumors happen to other people. This was something that was definitely not on my life's things-to-do list. After three years, I'm still coming to terms with it. And I can't say this enough, those have been the three longest years in my life. Much of what I went through during that time (the train rides to Long Beach and running at Wilson Track) are long ago a thing of the past to the point where it seems like it happened in another lifetime to someone else. I have to admit, the Lord sure filled up my life with something different and unusual. Nothing boring about the last three years.

It's late afternoon now. The sun is setting into a haze. The cat has been curled up in her bed most of the day. I've spent most of mine at my desk looking out at cloud shrouded mountains. It's very quiet and peaceful. Where do I go from here? More of the same adventures or has the time come to do something about what I just experienced. I've always believed that if I put my life in God's hands, I'll be where I'm supposed to be doing what He wants me to do. He made me feel most comfortable at my desk pecking away at my keyboard. He taught me lessons of faith. He's placed people in my life who were angels and inspiration. He's provided the companionship I need without the emotional overload that I didn't need. He's gently closed doors slowly enough that I would understand why. He's kept me safe, secure and fed and helped me realize what a blessing that is. Every time I felt down, He brought someone into my life who brought me back up. He's blessed me with talents that were always there and has made it possible for me to use them. He led me to a place where He wants me to be using those talents – writing, sharing the adventure of the last three years that He has blessed me with. I believe He wants me to write about that life and the story of that journey begins with the words,

"I was my smile."

THE END

December 3, 2010, 4:13 PM

David Douglas Shannon

In memory of Yikes

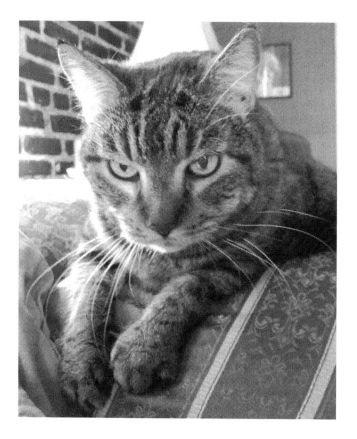

July 24, 1994 to May 31, 2011
Rest in peace, my little friend.

THE GLOSSARY

Other Stuff I Figured Out

OK, so that wasn't the actual end of the book. As usual, I have more to say. This is especially important for people who just discovered that they have an Acoustic Neuroma or people who are planning on getting one (you just never know). There is a bunch of medical stuff written about Acoustic Neuromas and surgery and possible negative outcomes. But that I've seen until now, they haven't been written by someone who has actually been through that crazy world firsthand. For the most part, it's been written by medical professionals who try to make it not sound so technical. They may know how to remove brain tumors but explaining things in simple terms is not one of their fortes. At least not in terms that I can fully understand. From my experience, most new ANer's I meet, have a lot of questions. Here are answers to some of those questions

The first question I usually get when I meet with a new ANer is, "Dave, what the heck is an Acoustic Neuroma?"

If I were to give you the medical explanation, I'd get a blank look sort of like you're thinking about what to have for dinner.

The simple Dave answer is that you have something like a cyst growing in your head that just keeps growing. Cysts grow all over the body. Most of them don't cause much trouble except mild discomfort and occasional pain. An AN doesn't even do that – unless, of course it gets too big (4 cm + is in the too big range – which by the way in Dave-talk is 1.6 inches +). Then all hell breaks loose. Actually, things could be worse. You could have an NF2 – a tumor a both sides of your head.

The second question I usually get is, "Dave, why did I get an Acoustic Neuroma?"

I'm sure there is a convoluted medical-speak explanation somewhere, but the simple answer is that you just had some bad luck. It is that simple. Although cell phone use has been rumored to be a cause, as of now, there is no evidence linking the two. Acoustic Neuromas after all, did exist before cell phones. Research also shows no genetic linkage – except in the case of an NF2.

Then there is the granddaddy of all questions spoken with a sense of doom, "Is an AN fatal?"

If it has been discovered, it isn't fatal so long as you care for it as your doctor suggests. If you allow it to continue to grow beyond "a watch and wait" period (which can be a prognosis with the smaller and slower growing tumors), then yes, it could be fatal or cause serious strokes. ANs are not malignant, meaning they don't produce cells that can travel to other parts of the body. They are benign. Now if you're one to look for sympathy, you don't have to tell anyone that. You can tell everyone in a solemn voice that you have a brain tumor followed by a look of pending doom.

Now there are those of you who haven't been diagnosed with an AN and are wondering how you'll know if you have one.

A doctor will tell you.

Oh, you mean what are the symptoms?

The most common initial symptoms are hearing loss, ringing in the ear (tinnitus) and dizziness and sudden loss of balance. As the tumor grows, other symptoms such as a fullness in the head, mental confusion, headaches and facial palsy may occur – which may lead to problems with swallowing and voice quality. If you have some of these symptoms, particularly the loss of balance and facial palsy, you might want to consider a trip to see an Otologist or an ENT. You'll probably need a referral from your primary care physician.

So you've been diagnosed with an Acoustic Neuroma and you're asking yourself "now what?"

You have several options and doing nothing is not one of them – although the first one may seem that way. The first is "watching and waiting." This may be suggested by your doctor. This occurs when the tumor is small, generally less than one centimeter. Over a period of time, you will have MRIs to determine the growth of the tumor. If it shows little growth, you may not need surgery. This is particularly true with the elderly where surgery may be too difficult for the patient and span of life is limited. It's a decision that you and your doctor will make together.

The second option, microsurgery, involves a hole in the head to remove the tumor. It's the most complex for the patient but it is the most thorough. There are three types of microsurgery. The first is a Translabyrinthine (more commonly known as a Translab). This procedure is used when the patient has little hearing that would need to be saved. It is the least complex (as brain surgery goes) and the most direct. The surgery plows directly through everything to get at the tumor. In the process it wipes out the hearing nerve, the balance nerve, and anything else that gets in the way. In my case, I was nearly deaf on the AN side, so I really wasn't losing much in the way of hearing. The second type of microsurgery is called a Retrosigmoid. (Retrosig for short). The surgeon enters three inches behind the ear. Through this procedure, hearing can sometimes be saved. The third microsurgery option is called a Middle-fossa (Mid-fossa). The surgeon enters the skull over the ear to get into and at the tumor. This procedure is used most often when the goal is to save the hearing nerve.

The third option to remove the tumor is through the use of

radiation. Radiation zaps the tumor into submission. This can be used when the tumor is small enough. The two radiology methods are CyberKnife (Deathray I) and Gamma Knife (Deathray II). (They aren't really called Deathrays – I just made that up). There are risks associated with radiation, including the possible failure to eradicate the tumor. Annual MRIs are necessary for life to determine possible re-growth. If you can't get enough MRIs, this could be the way to go.

Note: I have no intention of recommending any of these options. They are what they are and recommendations should only come from medical professionals. The final decision is made between you and your doctor.

Also note: When selecting a surgery team, choose one that specializes in Acoustic Neuroma surgery on a regular basis. This is no time for experimenting. Sorry, part-timers, but I'm looking out for my fellow ANers.

So, now that you've chosen one of the three options, you're probably wondering, what's next?

If you choose microsurgery, here's a laundry list of things you'll need to know for the "Big Dance."

1. It's expensive. Insurance will generally cover everything except co-pays and deductibles. But it's worth looking into just to make sure.
2. Everyone signs a Power of Attorney before surgery. Don't freak out.

3. The actual surgery lasts from four to six hours depending on the procedure for the surgical team. For those waiting for you in the waiting room, it will be several days. For you, it will be a second.

4. No matter how much you beg them not to, they'll shave the AN side of your head.

5. It doesn't hurt. You more than likely won't even feel the incision.

6. You will spend a day in ICU. After all, you just had a brain tumor removed, not tonsils.

7. There is an even chance that you will feel nauseous and vomit post-surgery. Nothing is wrong. You're just dealing with anesthesia and the loss of a balance nerve.

8. Some people experience headaches. Ouch. Request pain medicine – but avoid the number 10 stuff unless you're used to heroin.

9. If you have some facial paralysis, chances are your eye is going to hurt. Make sure you request and get eye lubricant. You probably will be wearing a moisture chamber over your eye.

10. Taste will be weird. It isn't the hospital food, although that may be a contributing factor.

11. You'll be thirsty post-surgery. They'll give you ice chips sparingly. You'll want more. They won't give them to you. You'll start an enemies list.

12. Plan on spending three to five days in the hospital. Your insurance company will want it to be three days. Your

doctor will want five. Your doctor will win.

13. Plan on walking the halls a lot whether you want to or not.

14. Your neck will probably be stiff and painful. After all, it was forced into a contorted position for several hours during surgery

15. You may notice an increase in your tinnitus if you have it.

16. You will have fat removed from your abdomen to plug up the hole in your head. (Seriously). You won't even notice it. Although "Fathead" will become an appropriate term for you.

17. The fat plug will be covered with titanium mesh. It won't set off metal detectors. "Metal Head" will also be appropriate.

18. You don't want to blow the hole in your head open. There are two obvious ways you can do this – blowing your nose too hard and exerting too strenuously when taking a bowel movement. Two things that will come in handy – nasal decongestants and laxatives.

19. You won't be allowed to wash your hair for several weeks after surgery. Sorry. You'll need to wear a bath cap if you want to take a shower. My advice to guys – get a "number one" cut – it'll grow back. And your hair length will always be one length.

20. You will be tired – very tired. Flash naps will occur, often lasting for a month (or at least seem that way).

21. Other than the normal stuff you'd take to the hospital like a tooth brush, toothpaste, deodorant and ladies and guy stuff, there are a few things that you'll need that no one ever tells you about (except me).

   - Lip balm. Including your pre-surgery fasting, you won't be allowed to drink water for about two days. You will be a bit dehydrated – so will your lips.
   - A pillow. If you're uncomfortable with strange pillows, you will be even more so with a sore neck.
   - Magazines or puzzles. Television won't make much sense to you as you drift in and out of sleep.
   - A laptop or a cell with an internet app. This is the easiest way to notify friends and family of your surgery outcome and it cuts down on phone calls that won't make much sense as you drift in and out of sleep.
   - Comfortable sweats or pajamas. You'll be taking frequent mandatory hall walks. Hospital gowns don't pass the modesty test.
   - Non-slip slippers. You may not have much balance during your hall walks and wearing slippery slippers only makes it worse.
   - Sunglasses. You could have some facial paralysis from mild to severe. In any case, you'll want to protect your eye as you leave the hospital. Direct sunlight feels like a needle being jabbed in your eye.
   - Medications that you normally take. Prior to entering

the hospital, check with your doctor to see what you should be taking and what might interfere with the medicines you'll be prescribed in the hospital.

- And lastly, a sense of humor. It's easier to deal with the prospect of talking out of the corner of you mouth like a pirate and staggering around like a drunk when viewed with humor.

22. You'll be sent home with a bunch of prescriptions. Get them filled immediately and begin taking them as directed. Be especially diligent with the steroids and any antibiotics as they are critical for healing.

23. You'll be sent home with a list of balance exercises. Do the exercises. In addition, have someone accompany you on walks for as long as you feel comfortable.

24. There could be a post-surgical issue called a CSF leak (cerebrospinal fluid). Generally this would happen in the hospital soon after surgery. But it could happen at home weeks, even months later. There is no blood in the brain, rather a clear liquid know as CSF. A leak shows itself generally by running from the nose or at the surgical incision. This needs to be taken care of immediately. Among other things, left uncared for, a leak could lead to Meningitis. According to the Journal of Otolaryngology (10/98) there is about a 20% risk of a CSF leak with a Translab and 15% chance with a Retosig.

25. Once you get through all this, you're still not out of the woods. ANs are pesky little critters. They sometimes grow back. Follow-up MRIs will be scheduled once about every three years.

That brings us to the third "what should I do about my AN" option, radiosurgery. In radiosurgery, specialized equipment zaps as many as 200 beams of radiation on the tumor. Generally, this procedure can be used for small tumors. Doctors may recommend this option because the patient isn't healthy enough for the demands of microsurgery or the patient may opt for this method because it's less invasive. The advantage of radiosurgery is that will do little or no damage to nerves surrounding the tumor.

If you chose this method or are considering it, here's what you need to know:

1. It's an outplacement visit that takes all day.

2. Most of the day you'll be walking around wearing a head-frame that has been attached to your head with four pins. Think of "Hellraiser" with a few less pins.

3. Once the helmet is in place, scans of the brain will be made to locate the tumor. This is probably a good idea.

4. During the actual procedure, you'll be lying on a bed with your head-frame attached to a helmet.

5. The procedure can take less than an hour up to four hours. This of course, will seem like days.

6. You won't feel the radiation. The tumor will, and no doubt scream for mercy.

7. After the surgery, you may feel some mild discomfort, but nothing like microsurgery.

8. You won't have the balance issues or hearing loss following microsurgery.

So this really sounds great – why don't more people opt for it. One of the reasons has been mentioned before – the tumor size has to be small. Usually, ANs are fairly big before the symptoms show up. There is also a downside to this. It takes 18 months to two years before the tumor cells have completely died off – and sometimes they don't. They could grow back. In microsurgery, the chances are that the tumor is history.

Now that you have the surgery out of the way and on the comeback trail, you're asking yourself, "Is this stuff finally over?"

Other than a tumor that springs back to life, there could be nothing that happens or there could be a bunch of things that happen. You read about four of them in my story. If you get through surgery successfully (meaning that you don't suffer from a rare stroke during the operation) there will be the three or four main issues that you could deal with. Or, in the majority of cases, nothing. In my case, as in the case of most post-surgery issues, the issues include balance, hearing loss, facial palsy, and cognitive disorder/disorientation.

Stemming from balance issues, the weird, wacky world of wonkyhead creeps up on many post-surgery ANers. The original temporary balance problems for some reason become permanent. Medical professionals scoff at its existence. They don't have it. Wonkyheads swear it exists. They have it. Like any surgery outcome, your mileage may vary. Some miss it entirely. Others deal with it to various degrees – sometimes continuously like I do. Because the medical world tends to ignore it, there is little research and is subject to passing smirks.

So being a curious wonkyhead, here's some of the stuff that I figured out talking to fellow wonkies and those without it. It seems that two things factor into its existence. One is the size of the tumor and the other is vestibular therapy.

There is an AN microsurgery given – you're going to lose you balance nerve on the AN side. There is no way around it. As I mentioned in my story, technically the balance nerve on the non-AN side should compensate and make everything cool. Technically. Now here's what I think happens. Pre-surgery ANers with large tumors (three+ cms, 1.2 inches in Dave-talk) are already experiencing balance loss problems because the larger tumor has already grown to the size that it is messing around with the balance nerve. Over time, as the tumor grows, the nerve on the opposite side gradually compensates. By the time surgery rolls around, the nerve on the good side has already figured things out and is ready to take over. Those with smaller tumors, however, haven't experienced a balance loss severe enough that the nerve on the other side has yet to learn anything. So when surgery comes along, it's business as usual. But after surgery it's whammo, a crash course in balance – no gradual learning time.

As I mentioned in my story, there are three components of balance -- the leg and spine sensors, vision, and the inner ear. If one of the three is messed with, the remaining two come to the rescue – sort of. If leg coordination is good and vision is good, the brain figures a way to compensate and skips the inner ear system, settling on the other two to get by. Because of that, the remaining balance nerve is never forced to adapt. And this is where wonkyhead comes from. Balance is questionable when it's just relying on just two legs of a three legged stool. It's almost hopeless when it's down to one leg. What would cause that? Disruptions to vision could. In a normal, sedentary position (sitting or standing) where vision is stable and precise, wonkyhead doesn't exist. But when the body goes into motion and vision and the leg and spine sensory system are put to the test, wonkyhead rears it pesky little…well, head. Vision is disrupted by motion and other stimulus. The greater the motion, as in running or riding in a car that is bouncing around, the greater the wonkyhead because vision has a difficult time focusing in order to send balance signals to the brain. The resulting sensation is that the brain feels like it is bouncing inside the head or the head feels like a fishbowl with water sloshing around inside. In reality, it's the vision that is sending mixed messages and the brain isn't catching on. Something as simple as turning your head while walking throws the balance system into chaos because the eyes are not focusing on the business of maintaining balance.

One thing I'd like to mention. I used the term wonkyhead quite a bit in this last passage. It sounds silly. The term may be, but the condition isn't. I'm always open to a more clinical sounding name (as long as it isn't Latin and can be pronounced by an average human). It's just that the folks on the ANA forum came up with a name that describes the condition so well.

So what can be done to correct this balance issue post-surgery? Immediate, intensive, and intrusive vestibular therapy is needed. In my case, I was sent home with a list of balance exercises. I did them, but not with the passion that was needed because I didn't understand the balance system. It wasn't until I enlisted in a balance boot camp six months later that I recognized the need for rigorous training. By then, I was on the road to too late. Over the past four years, my balance has either improved or I'm getting used to it being messed up. Again – "the new normal."

Here's what I think should be done. For those with smaller tumors (under 2.5 cm) vestibular training should begin prior to surgery. This way the future remaining nerve has already begun the process of adapting by the time surgery rolls around. Now I'm not a scientist or a medical professional or a vestibular therapist, but the way I see things – it makes sense. And too, what do you have to lose by taking a few steps of preparation. If your insurance allows, you could see a vestibular therapist. Short of that, on the next page is a list of vestibular training exercises that I've gathered over the years. They are geared toward a concentrated learning process for the remaining nerve. One caution. Since most of these exercises could severely throw you off balance, make sure to follow the safety precautions that are given with every exercise.

VESTIBULAR TRAINING EXCERSISES

1. Walking. It sounds simple but it works. Immediately after surgery and in the early days after, take frequent walks with someone to assist you if needed. While walking, look from side to side. You may feel dizzy (the reason to do this with someone), but repeat it as frequently as is comfortable.

2. In an open area inside without obstructions that you could fall into, do the heel-to-toe walk (drunk test). Walk back and forth across the area several times until you feel comfortable. Then try it with your eyes closed. This may take some time to adjust to it.

3. Stand on one leg with your eyes open as long as you are able. Then try it with your eyes closed (this is difficult under normal circumstances).

4. Place a chair or sofa cushion in the corner of a room. This needs to be in a corner so that if you lose your balance you can catch yourself against one of the walls. Stand on the cushion with your feet slightly apart. Close your eyes and stand there without moving for three minutes. If it is too difficult, move your feet farther apart. As you adjust to the exercise over time, move your feet closer together as you stand.

5. While standing on the cushion in the corner, focus your eyes on an object in the room. While keeping your eyes focused ahead, move your head back and forth slowly as if you are saying "no."

These are some exercises to get you started. If balance problems persist, you may need to see a vestibular therapist. Again, safety is the most important consideration. Don't push yourself to the point of falling.

Up next on the list of things that could go annoyingly wrong, is hearing loss. Chances are that you will be deaf in the AN ear. Many ANers have already been dealing with tinnitus in that ear already and possibly a slight loss of hearing and may be accustomed to it. Single-sided deafness or SSD is difficult but not impossible. You will have to make adjustments – like where to sit at a tableful of people to hear the maximum conversation, like where to sit in a movie theater, like increasing the use of the words uh, what, pardon and again, like getting use to the lack of stereo when listening to music through headphones, like missing entire conversations because someone was prattling on next to your deaf side and you weren't aware of it. It does have its advantages though. To block out noise while trying to sleep at night, all one has to do is sleep on their good ear. It's also a good excuse for doing something wrong as in "Oh, I must not have heard you."

There are solutions for this beyond ASL and lip-reading that I will get to in a moment. But something needs to be said that should go without saying that needs to be written in capital letters. PROTECT THE HEARING IN YOUR GOOD EAR! It's all that stands between you and total deafness. Here are some cautions and taboos:

1. No more loud concerts. None. Without earplugs. I assure you that the musicians on stage are wearing them.

2. If you're listening to music through headsets or earbuds and you can't hear someone who is talking to you, the volume is too loud. The days of ear-splitting rock n' roll are over.

3. No more operating machinery like lawnmowers or

power tools without earplugs. When in doubt, err on
the side of caution – wear the earplugs.

4. If attending a motor sports event – wear earplugs –
especially open-wheel Indy-car type races.

5. Cover your ear or close the car windows around police,
fire truck, or ambulance sirens.

6. Keep your ear canal clean to prevent infections.

7. Don't stick any objects in your ear that could puncture
your eardrum.

8. Use common sense…or learn ASL.

There are situations, particularly in loud enclosed places like
restaurants and clubs, where hearing even on a normal level is difficult.
In any situation like that, there are tricks to get others to speak up. When
greeting someone, greet them in the volume in which you wish to carry
on the conversation. More than likely, they will respond at the same
volume. There are of course mumblers and what I call "small-talkers,"
who no matter how many times you say "what" will continue on at their
miniscule speaking levels. In my experience, I've found that if it gets
to a point of frustration, remind the person that you are partially deaf.
If they continue, move on with an "I am sorry, I just can't hear you." I
designed a T-shirt for situations like that. It looks like this:

My hearing loss is a disability. Your mumbling isn't.

SPEAK UP!

http://www.cafepress.com/britanniak

Now what you've been waiting for -- the good news. Something can be done to counter SSD. If you have relatively good hearing in your "good ear" and have a cooperative insurance company, you could be a candidate for a BAHA. BAHA stands for bone-anchored hearing aid. It's a device that is surgically implanted in the skull (seriously) which transmits sound through the bone to the inner ear on the good side. A three millimeter hole (.1 inches) is drilled into the skull and an abutment is implanted into the bone. A sound processor is attached to the abutment. I'm not making this up. It does look a bit Frankensteinish but hair easily covers it. However, a warning to a hair stylist in advance would certainly be in order. Those that I know who wear them, swear by them.

The procedure takes a few hours. It's done as an outpatient generally sometime after AN surgery. However, I believe I have heard of some instances where the abutment was implanted during the hospital stay immediately following the surgery.

One other potential surgery downside that I haven't mentioned is tinnitus. Most ANers are already dealing with it at some level and have become adjusted to it. I've had it for 25 years and I really don't even notice it until I'm thinking about it – like now. There was at least one case that I know of, however, where surgery made the tinnitus worse to the point where the individual had another surgery to attempt to correct it. Generally, there is no cure for tinnitus. Some research has indicated that it can become worse from smoking, drinking alcohol, loud noises, and stimulants like coffee. One doctor indicated to me that some research has shown that Melatonin reduces the volume – although I have seen nothing further on the study. Unfortunately, tinnitus is one of those annoyances that one has to live with.

Which brings up another annoyance – a big one – and a byproduct of AN surgery – facial palsy and its partner in crime, Synkinesis. I really don't know what the probability of ending up with either is. Early on in the pre-surgery process, I believe I was told the chances for facial paralysis were 1 to 5% percent. I've read it's 10 to 15 %. I don't know that there is a viable estimate. I'm under the impression that no one keeps track of these things and most people are just making some wild guess. It does happen though and as an AN patient you need to be aware of the possibility. Here's what you need to know.

The facial nerve is bunched in there with the other cranial nerves that are associated with an Acoustic Neuroma. While the chances of it being severed are probably pretty low, the opportunity for it to be aggravated are probably pretty good – especially when it comes to the larger tumors. In my case, the tumor had grown onto the nerve and when the sticky tumor was pulled off, it stretched the nerve. The stretched nerve didn't like that and went into dormancy. Unfortunately, surgeons don't know what nerves the tumor is affecting until they get a first-hand look at the thing. I have heard of situations where the patient requested that if the tumor had grown onto the facial nerve to merely have it cut and leave the remaining part on the nerve without irritating the nerve. Then, at a later time, the remaining part of the tumor would be zapped with radiation. I knew of one young woman who opted for that approach but I lost track of her to learn of the outcome.

So here's the deal. Based on a lot of stuff I've read and heard (no, I can't attribute one source), if during surgery your facial nerve has been messed with, and if you wake up from surgery with facial paralysis, and you leave the hospital with facial paralysis, you may be dealing with it for some time. Again, the prognoses for its duration are all over the board. Some say weeks. Some say months. Some say a year. And that could be as random as it actually is. Mine actually lasted for about three months until the nerves that came back to life chose to rewire wrong causing Synkinesis (good going, nerves). In any case, no matter what the duration, there are some immediate concerns which need to be addressed.

The first issue is the eye. This is where you can run into big trouble. Facial paralysis generally means you won't get full eye closure. As a result, since it is constantly exposed to air, it will become dry and painful. That's bad enough. But there's a real danger in this. A dry cornea could lead to serious eye damage. It is critical that you keep your eye lubricated with eye lubricant and that you are in the care of an ophthalmologist. Most of the issues regarding facial paralysis are more cosmetic and less pressing. The eye is a critical issue.

There are surgical procedures to enhance the blink in the eye. One is to have small gold or platinum weights placed in the upper eyelid. There are also sticker weights that are less intensive than surgery, but less effective as well. In some of the more serious cases, a tiny spring is placed in the corner of the eye which facilitates blinking. Cauterization of the tear duct is another option. Success for these procedures varies. I know of one person where this didn't work at all and she continues to suffer from dry eye issues. I should also mention that I have heard from some physical therapists and surgeons that it is better to allow the eye to regain movement through non-surgical means rather that mechanical means.

Another negative side effect of facial paralysis involves dental issues. With paralysis comes tightening of the face, particularly the cheek. The cheek presses hard on the teeth preventing the normal flow of saliva which would naturally remove trapped food particles. It is critical that extra care be given to daily dental hygiene as well as regular cleanings by a dentist. Infections could occur which endanger the health of the teeth and gums.

While the ability to smile is the least health concern, it is obviously an emotional, cosmetic issue. A smile is a critical non-verbal communication device. Those with palsy may find themselves being self-conscious about the ability to manage only a one-sided smile and rely on a closed mouth grin (as I usually find myself doing). For some, this can be devastating.

I really sympathize with those of you who are – it ended my career – I understand. But my advice to you, it's best to accept who you are now. You can be angry. You can be frustrated. You can be hurt. But that's not going to solve things.

There is hope for you who are dealing with facial palsy. Through physical therapy and home exercises, the tightness associated with palsy can be alleviated to a degree providing whatever smile the nerve action will allow.

One treatment that has been sternly nixed is that of electric stimulation of the nerves to jolt them back to life. I don't know why it isn't viable, but everyone I talked with was pretty emphatic about not doing it.

Palsy management requires a strong degree of dedication and desire. Home facial exercises are a must. Hot pad, massage, and facial movement should be part of an every day routine. Massage by a Physical Therapist should be regular – once a month or as insurance coverage allows. Without that, tightness in the face will increase and elasticity will be lost.

I should also mention that facial reanimation therapy is a specialty. There isn't a physical therapist who deals with facial reanimation in every city and town. While I've made it a practice in this book not to recommend any specific medical providers, I'm going to make an exception here. I will give the names of three specialists to help guide you in the right direction. While I am sure there are others out there, I can only vouch for the positive results that I've heard from these three. They are:

David Douglas Shannon

Jackie Diels	Madison, Wisconsin
Teresa England	Garden Grove, California
Wanda Crook	San Diego, California

Likewise, there are others who I have heard of that produced less than stellar results. They won't be named. It goes without saying, however, check their credentials when enlisting the services of a physical therapist who specializes in facial re-animation.

There are also numerous facial exercise lists. The Bell's Palsy website has one such list. I, however, am not including any exercises. Facial re-animation is a technical, neuro-muscular effort and exercises should first be taught by a therapist who can analyze your particular needs. I'd also like to mention that the Bell's Palsy website (www.bellspalsy.ws) has a wealth of information on facial paralysis that goes into far more depth than I've gone into. For the most part, it's a good, easy read.

Again, there are more estimates for recovery than I can count. It seems like two years is the magic number. If your face hasn't returned to the old normal by then, they say it won't get any better. That is, of course, what "they" say. There are several palsy success stories on the Acoustic Neuroma Association forum. One individual posted her yearly smile progression. The improvement over four years was incredible. What was once an obvious drawn down corner of the mouth is back to nearly normal with a nearly normal smile. I believe desire and determination has a lot to do with success and less to do with time.

There are some other recent advances for the more severe cases of facial palsy where there is a pronounced draw-down at the corner of the mouth. A relatively new procedure called a Temporalis Tendon Transfer (a T-3 for short) has been developed at Johns Hopkins University Hospital in Baltimore. Now what I can figure from what I've been told and read, a tendon is taken from the leg or the head or the cheek (this part is actually a bit confusing) and reattached to the corner of the mouth. As a result, when the face is at rest, the mouth is more symmetrical and natural looking. Kay and Nancy, two ladies on the Acoustic Neuroma Association forum, have both had the T-3 and love the results. The procedure itself is relatively short at about 90 minutes – the recovery and muscle retraining is a bit longer.

There's another procedure – it's a mouthful – called a Hypoglossal-facial nerve interpositional – jump graft. Just saying it lulls me into a catatonic stupor. Fortunately, it is simply referred to as a 12-7 Jump. In this procedure, the 12th cranial nerve (it's up there with those balance and hearing nerves) that controls the tongue is connected to the facial nerve (the 7th cranial nerve) that has been playing dead since surgery. The thinking is that active movement of the tongue stimulates the 12th nerve which in turn by its activity encourages the 7th nerve to join the world again – sort of a nerve to nerve "hey bud, let's party." Who thinks this stuff up?

Now if you end up with Synkinesis, there is good news and bad news. The good news is that the facial nerves that were messed with during surgery have finally decided to cooperate. The bad news is that for some reason, they rewired wrong. You'll have facial movement but it won't be normal. And unfortunately, the damage has been done.

There is no magic cure for Synkinesis. However, it can be managed. I briefly covered all that in my story. Synkinesis is the involuntary muscle reaction to a voluntary muscle movement. The eye blinks voluntarily which causes the corner of the mouth to pull up involuntarily. The lips attempt to move up into a smile while rogue neck muscles try to pull it down. But through a combination of Botox, physical therapy, and home exercises, the effects of Synkinesis can be held to a minimum. Botox freezes the muscles that are creating the havoc. Physical Therapy relaxes the face so that the muscles can be re-animated. And home exercise increases that retraining. From my experience, and that of others, it works. The Synkinesis won't go away and there will always be subtle indications like the arch of an eyebrow, but with therapy, it's hardly noticable to anyone. Until you of course attempt a smile --- dead giveaway.

While Botox may seem like an extravagant cosmetic procedure that couldn't possibly be covered by insurance, for Synkinesis it is coded as a neurological procedure and generally covered. Since Synkinesis is a permanent thing, the treatment is too, as long as you want to keep the facial tightness under some sort of control. But do note, it does take a regular regime of all three programs – Botox, physical therapy and home exercise – to make it work. Personally, I've gone back and forth with treatment and haven't always been diligent. Then, as has actually happened, I yawn and can't get my mouth closed so I hustle my way back to PT. For others, it's the eye issues that keep them involved.

That pretty much sums up the big three negative AN surgery outcomes. In most cases, hearing loss is a given. SSD is annoying but manageable. Balance issues are common but can be dealt with. Facial Palsy, while not necessarily that frequent is still a bit to deal with when it occurs.

Now you probably don't want to hear this, but there are more post-surgery complications. Two of them are important enough that the Acoustic Neuroma Association devotes separate discussion categories to each on the Forum.

The first of these categories is Cognitive and Emotional Issues. I mentioned this in passing in my story. From what I've read, cognitive issues include short-term memory loss, the inability to concentrate, speech difficulties, and IQ loss among others. I've also read in numerous Blogs and newsletters that doctors seem to dismiss this much as they do wonkyhead. Why, I don't know. Seems to me that if it's enough of an issue that it pops up a bunch on Google searches and that the ANA is aware of it, it should receive some attention.

There are a number of factors that could potentially contribute to cognitive difficulties. One of the immediate factors is that of prolonged anesthesia. Somewhere along the line, it doesn't seem as though the brain would act favorably to being knocked out for five to six hours. I would imagine that it is similar to that of a punch-drunk boxer. Similarly, in some AN surgical procedures, the brain is moved. I also got to believe that the king of the body is not going to be cool with that. These seem to be short-term issues.

Personally, I've experienced some of them. I used to sprint (even as an old guy). I can't anymore. I used to play the keyboards pre-surgery. Now I struggle. I used to have excellent handwriting. Now it's more like chicken-scratching. But more than anything, it's my speech that seems to have been affected. Pre-surgery, I spoke very clearly and was never at a loss for words or wit. Today I struggle with articulating thoughts. Others have mentioned the same thing. Several folks have suggested that the brain is over-working as it focuses on hearing and balance loss issues and that bit of multi-tasking leaves cognitive thought in the lurch. I'll buy that.

The other part of the Forum category is Emotional. Everyone is going to deal with the AN nasties in his or her own way. From the tumor discovery to post-surgery recovery, it's a bumpy and chaotic ride. As I said in my story in the beginning of this book, others have accepted my fate for me and have moved on. I'm sure that happens quite a bit to others and we are left to fend in our personal struggles alone. While looking at the ANA forum the other day under the Cognitive/Emotional Issues category, I saw a post that started off "I'm ready to throw in the towel." I panicked at first thinking they were ready to throw in the life towel. I read on and realized that they were expressing their frustration with post-surgery care, the lack of results, and the run-around they were experiencing.

There were other posts that day. Depression. Anger. Resentment. Loneliness. Resignation. Exhaustion. If you're an AN postie and you feel you're alone in dealing with these issues, you're not. You have company – lots of it. Outside seeking professional help in the most severe cases, I've found that misery loves company and that it goes a long way in coping. You are different post-surgery – particularly if you are dealing with a less than stellar recovery. Whether you wanted to or not, you've joined an elite club.

The Acoustic Neuroma Association provides an opportunity to share feelings and frustrations which helps you realize that you're not alone. In addition to the Forum, the ANA organizes local support groups in many cities across the country which allow AN posties to share in a face-to-face setting. There are also several Facebook AN groups. If friends and family don't seem to understand (note to friends and family who are reading this, please understand) look into the ANA forum and ANA support groups.

To pass along a personal experience on this emotional issue, when I told someone that my Synkinesis was permanent just after I got the news, she blankly looked at me and said "I wonder if it's too early to get my winter purses out."

It was like getting hit in the face with a slushball. I realized then that there are a mess of emotions that many ANer's deal with that are invisible to the impervious outside world. As I read posts on the Forum, the Cognitive/Emotional Issues category seems to be the most confusing and the least understood. There doesn't seem to be any meaningful research into it nor does there seem to be a pattern of support.

The second of the non-traditional categories on the ANA Forum is that of Headaches. This is easily the most debilitating of those post-surgery consequences. I'm just not going to do it justice because I don't have any post-surgery issues with headaches or pain. To this point, everything I've written has been personal experience. I only know what I've been told and what I've read by those who have the misfortune of dealing with it. And what I've read has been both heart-wrenching as it is confusing.

The causes and the treatments seem to be all over the board. The potential causes range from the movement of the cerebellum during Retro-Sig surgery, to nerves growing into the titanium mesh covering the surgical hole in the head, to just a complete mystery. And for all the potential causes, there are just as many suggested treatment options. There is the traditional drug route, the pain management specialists route, the acupuncture route, and one called a myofacial release (which sounds a bit like facial massage for Synkinesis) among others.

Associated with headaches is that of facial pain. This can generally be traced back to the fifth cranial nerve called the nervus trigeminus. It's also right up there with the balance, facial and hearing nerves. While not immediately in the path of nerve destruction, if trifled with it can cause facial pain known as trigeminal neuralgia. Although this happens less often, I know of several posties who deal with it.

And while we're on the subject of cranial nerves, there are two others that should be mentioned that don't get much attention. They are the 9th and 10th cranial nerves. When they are annoyed, it's possible that swallowing becomes difficult and that there are taste disturbances on the rear third of the tongue. Theoretically, the back part of the tongue senses bitter tastes with salty tastes immediately preceding that on the tongue (some disagree with that).

From personal experience, intense taste disturbance crops up immediately after surgery and hangs around for a couple of months or so until returning to somewhat normal. I say somewhat normal because I still add Tabasco Sauce to most everything I eat to taste anything. And I do have problems swallowing pills that I never had before. But, of all the post-surgery issues you could encounter, unless you're in a culinary profession, these seem to be the least of the problems. I should also mention that when the 9th cranial nerve is provoked, posties will notice a metallic taste in their mouth for a few weeks. This seems to happen fairly frequently. It eventually goes away.

OK, that's it – no more bad news. Of course, I do hate to be the one to break this stuff to you, but you sure aren't going to hear most of it from anyone else. Why you won't – I don't know. Maybe because the medical professionals don't want to send you running. Maybe because they discount the consequences. Maybe because they're not concerned (which I certainly hope isn't the case). Or maybe because they know the odds are in their favor. But according to the Gale Encyclopedia of Cancer, approximately 20% of Acoustic Neuroma patients will experience some degree of post-surgery complications. Now whether that includes a stiff neck or taste disturbance, I don't know. But I do know stuff does happen.

I should point out that I've drawn some conclusions and have made some inferences that many not necessarily be accurate. When you spend months researching scientific terminology and practices and you can't stand science to begin with – especially 12- syllable Latin terms, one tends to go brain dead and could mess up. But for all the professional eye-rolling I may get, I have one perspective that gives me a bit of a leg up. I experienced this thing first hand. I live in my skin. They learn their stuff second-hand.

If you've recently discovered that you have an Acoustic Neuroma, you're setting out on a capricious adventure. Unless something happens drastic during surgery (as it could during any surgery), you will survive. But prepare yourself for some potential changes. You may experience nothing but fatigue and dizziness, but go into this thing with your eyes open.

If you are a friend or family of a newly diagnosed ANer, please be understanding and patient. They'll need you and your support – maybe for a long time. This isn't a sprained wrist, it's brain surgery. And that

ANer friend or family member of yours may come out on the post-surgery side as a different person – not a different personality, but as a person who sees things differently, who experiences things in a different way, who carries something within their heart and thoughts that they can't express.

By the way, I do know of some husbands who left their very beautiful crooked-smiling wives. To them – in the politest of terms I can muster – I say "Screw you." But for every one of them, there are so many more who have been faithful and supportive and to them, on behalf of this very exclusive club of ANer's, I say, "Thank you." There are a bunch of you I don't know, but for the ones that I do, thank you Dave, Hunter, Phil, James, Malcolm, Greg, Willie, Mike, Louie, Paul, Truman, Dexter, Jim and Joseph (Lord knows I'm missing someone). And for those of you ladies who have been dealing with us AN guys – thank you too. We can be a handful.

Well, I guess that's all I had to say. It's been an amazing journey. With all the setbacks along the way, I still wouldn't trade it for the world – though it does wear me out just thinking and writing about it. For those of you who are approaching a surgery date, rock n' roll! And for all of you, may God bless you with peace and a life full of happiness, love, and very cool things.

David Shannon

FAMOUS PEOPLE WITH ACOUSTIC NEUROMAS

Mark Ruffalo Actor, Director, Writer. Mark has starred in movies such as *The Kids are All Right, Eternal Sunshine of the Spotless Mind, Shutter Island,* and *Zodiac.* His AN surgery was in early 2002. He had complications with facial paralysis, balance, and cognitive thinking. In an interview in *New York Magazine*, he admitted that he even had a hard time remembering how to tie knots. His recovery has been complete. On a personal note, I met Mark on the set of *Zodiac* while I was working as a stand-in in 2006. Little did I realize that I would be facing the same issues that he did a year later.

Tionne Watkins Singer. Tionne (Tboz) was a member of the 90's Hip-Hop girl group, TLC. TLC had hits such as "Waterfalls," "Diggin' on You," and "Unpretty." She had her surgery in November 2006. Her complications were balance, facial paralysis, and hearing.

Dusty Hill Singer, bassist. Dusty is a member of the Texas Blues/ Rock band, ZZ Top. ZZ Top is known for hits such as "Sharp Dressed Man," "Legs," and "Give Me All Your Lovin'." He was diagnosed with an AN in early 2007 which forced the cancellation of a tour as he was being treated.

ACKNOWLEDGEMENTS

This has been a very long, often bone-jarring, ride. As I have mentioned many times, just reliving it through writing about it has been exhausting. This is sort of a bittersweet ending to a period of my life as I package it up and move on to another adventure. There were, of course, the ugly moments. But there were so many more blessed memories that I want to savor over and over again as if they were happening for the first time. I can't. That's what makes it so bittersweet. I started the journey younger and innocent and ended older and wiser, which is probably the way things should work out. I had help along the way – a lot of it. In closing, I want to thank those who shared this adventure with me and helped me along the way. I will forever be grateful for what you did for me.

I would first like to thank the Acoustic Neuroma Association and the ANA Forum members without whom I'd still be stumbling around in the dark without a clue of what was happening to me. You are my family.

There are many friend and family members I want to thank, but first I'd like to express my sincere thanks and indebtedness to two people who I have never had the opportunity to meet but who had a profound impact on my life. The first is to Stacy Jackson of the SAG Foundation and to the Foundation itself. Without their support I would never have been able to continue my very much needed physical therapy after surgery.

The second thanks goes to Karen Wiener and the Will Rogers Motion Picture Pioneers Foundation. Without their support I would never have been able to afford the hearing aid for my "good" ear – which without that, I would be for the most part totally deaf.

Next on the thank-you list are the financial angels. Not many realized how desperate things were for me in my early days post-surgery. I was told I would be fine and able to return to work no more than two months after surgery. That's how I planned it. It would be tough financially on the very lean State Disability payments (especially when they were held up by the clinic), but I would squeak by. When that two months ended and I wasn't able to return to work, I was living on peanut butter and tap water while watching my world slowly crumble around me. These angels held it together.

Donna Leavy

Rick and Nancy Shannon (who also provided a much needed getaway place in Hawaii)

Dani Pedlow

Cindy Meadows

Next were those who provided moral support. Things were grim early on. I was lonely. I was uncertain. I was drifting without any focus. These folks kept me motivated with their companionship and concern.

James and Tracie Groh

Jessica Pappas

David Douglas Shannon

Steve Harding (my Christian rock in the storm)
Cindy Meadows (a repeat performance on thank you's)
Cheri Wood (my Christian sister)

Next on the thank you list was the one who kept me moving forward, always presenting challenges whether they be running, exercise, golf, kayaking, or assisting in business planning all while not letting me slip into self-pity. She gave me goals and a purpose in life.

Britannia Kathleen Shannon (my daughter)

During the first two years and especially during the first few critical months, I was unable to drive and had to rely on public transportation for follow-up medical and physical therapy appointments as best as I was able. But it wasn't always possible. These folks gave up their time and made sure I got to the appointments.

Freddy Hernandez
Justin Alvarez
Linda Harcharic

Then there is a thanks to one person who checked up on me every week. It may have only been through emails but there were spans of solitude when it felt good to know there was someone who was concerned.

Suzie Lauer

Hell in the Head

One of the toughest parts of writing this book was a concern whether this was actually interesting to anyone beside me. I needed readers to tell me. Unfortunately, no one seemed to have the time – except for one person – my best critic.

Bonnie Meadows

Next I owe a big thanks to my partners in crime. They kept me grounded. They understood what I was dealing with because they had gone through it as well.

Lanie Adams

Nancy Yaldizian

Next, of all things, are my Facebook friends. Some of them are AN survivors, a few are ex-girlfriends, folks from the acting business, friends from the long ago past, and some people I don't even know except as friends of friends. I don't hear well. It's hard for me to socialize in public. And I really don't have a lot of opportunity to get together with others. These friends actually gave me a social life – as two dimensional as it was – but I felt like I was involved with lives other than mine.

Then there was someone who was touching my life in a powerful way...and he didn't know it. I was a regular churchgoer. It ended though when, due to my poor hearing, I could no longer understand the messages. I have to be close enough to read lips. Some clown standing on stage in front of the minister just wasn't going to cut it. Then I found it. Andy Stanley, Senior Pastor of North Point Community Church in Atlanta, was broadcasting his messages on the internet – a week later but

170

in terms of eternity, what's a week. I had attended North Point when I lived in Atlanta and it felt like I was home watching Andy and guest speakers. I began to make a point to tune in every Sunday morning – before football games. Those messages saw me through some pretty rugged times.

Finally there are the two who inspire me, one through her amazing heart and compassion and the other through her unbreakable spirit. Whenever I felt down, whenever I felt there was no where to turn, whenever I began to feel self-pity and start to dwell on all that was bad in my life, I looked to these incredibly beautiful woman and I realized just how fortunate I was to have them in my life. Their strength gave me my strength. Both of you don't know how much you meant to me. I wrote this book for you.

Angie McMillan

Beth Reed

I thank you all. It's been great having you along sharing this incredible adventure with me. I don't know what I would have done without each of you.

Most importantly, I give my thanks to my Lord God. Without Him, I would not have appreciated the beauty of this journey. Without Him, I would be wallowing in fear and doubt (the other hell in the head). Without His love and guidance, I would be lost. God blessed me with this crazy adventure and helped me realize just how fortunate I was to live it and to share it with you. I praise Him and thank Him.

REFERENCES AND LINKS

References

Acoustic Neuroma Association, "Basic Overview," Cumming, GA, Feb. 2010

Mayo Foundation (MFMER), "What is an Acoustic Neuroma," Sept. 2010

California Ear Institute, "Acoustic Neuroma," Palo Alto, CA, Nov. 2011

T. Hain, "Acoustic Neuroma," Chicago Dizziness and Hearing, Northwestern University, Dec. 2011

G. Vyas, S. Voidya, A. Sharma, "World Articles on Ear, Nose and Throat," Vol. 3-1, 2010

Mayo Foundation (MFMER), "Gamma-knife Surgery," Oct. 2010

House Ear Clinic, "Hearing Impairment: Practical Suggestions for the Patient and Family," #35, Rev. Aug. 2005

University of Maryland Medical Center, Center for Auditory Solutions, "What is a BAHA?" Baltimore MD, 2011

B. Kovacsovics, L. Davidson, H.Hender, B. Magnuson, T. Ledin, The

International Tinnitus Journal, Vol. 4 No. 1, Jan. 1998

R. Ruben, "Hearing Loss and Deafness," The Merck Manual, Whitehouse Station, N.J., Apr. 2007

American Speech – Language – Hearing Association, "Causes of Hearing Loss in Adults," 2011

The House Clinic, "Auditory Brainstem Implants," Los Angeles, CA, 2011

T. England, "Current Concepts in Rehabilitation of Balance and Vestibular Disorders," ANA Notes, Issue 90, June 2004

Susan Herdman, "Vestibular Rehabilitation," F. A. David Company, Jan. 2000

L. Vereeck, F. L. Wuyts, S. Truijen, C. Valck, P. H. van de Heyning, "The Effects of Early Customized Vestibular Rehabilitation on Balance After Acoustic Neuroma Resection," Department of Health Sciences, University College of Antwerp, Merksum, Belgium, Aug, 2008.

Brainport Technologies, Wicab Inc. Middleton, WI, 2011

Acoustic Neuroma Association, "Facial Nerve and Acoustic Neuroma – Possible Damage and Rehabilitation," Cumming, GA, July 2010

The Facial Paralysis Institute, "Synkinesis," Beverly Hills, CA, May 2009

T. Cross, C. Sheard, P. Garrud, T. Nikolopoulos, G. O'Donoghue, "The Impact of Facial Paralysis on Patients with Acoustic Neuroma," The Laryngoscope, Volume 110, Issue 9, Jan. 2009

Journal of Otolaryngology, "CSF Leak" Oct. 1998

Michigan Ear Institute, "Acoustic Neuroma – Taste Disturbance and Mouth Dryness," Farmington Hills, MI, Rev. Dec. 2010

B. Bigelow, K. Edgar, "Encyclopedia of Drugs and Addictive Substances," Dec. 2005

Doughty, "Hawaii, The Big Island Revealed," Wizard Publications, 2010.

T. Gale, J. Lange, "The Gale Encyclopedia of Cancer," Gale Publishing, Nov. 2005

Links

While the preceding references provide some valuable reading if you have the time to wade through them, here are some great links for quick information.

For the most comprehensive, non-biased information on Acoustic Neuromas, turn to the Acoustic Neuroma Association. While there are other information sources, they may tend to slant their approach to selling products and services (a bit cynical, but what I've noticed). The ANA is a non-profit organization which provides valuable insight, support, and services to the AN community.

www.anausa.org

Associated with the ANA is the ANA Discussion Forum. It is a forum for AN patients and caregivers. Pre and post surgery patients are able to ask questions, answer questions, impart wisdom, share experiences, and join the company of other individuals facing the same issues that they are. It costs nothing to join and if you aren't interested in participation, you need not register to read the posts. The following is a list of Forum discussion topics:

AN Issues	Pretreatment Options	Eye Issues
Inquiries	Microsurgical Options	Cognitive/Emotional
Hearing Issues	Radiosurgical Options	Physicians
Insurance	Headaches	Caregivers
NF2	Facial Issues	AN Community
Watch and Wait	Balance Issues	Local Support Groups

www.anausa.org/smf/index.php

Ever want to share with someone what your tinnitus sounds like? Here's a link that mimics the various sounds. There's a good chance yours is included.

www.ata.org/sounds-of-tinnitus

The ANA did a survey in 1998 to determine what long-term affects were for members who underwent surgical and radiosurgical procedures. While the survey is a bit old and there have been some advances in post-surgical care, this is at least an indicator and an easy read.

www.dinagoldin.com/anarchive/life.htm

If the last site is an easy read, this one is just the opposite. This link is a cumbersome beast of a survey done by the ANA in 2007. By cumbersome, I mean 75 pages worth. I fell asleep after 21 of them – and as a former marketing guy, I was used to this stuff. But if you're a raw data statistics-type, this will be right up there with your all-time favorite links.

www.anausa.org/index.php/patient-survey-2007-2008?tmp/=component&format=raw

If you are an AN patient who's looking at microsurgery, there is a chance you could experience some sort of facial paralysis (whatever that chance may be). While I did go into it in my simplified way, The Bell's Palsy site has a wealth of information told in an easy to understand style about a very complex subject. Even I understood most of it until of course they started using those pesky Latin medical terms.

www.bellspalsy.ws/

While I'm on the subject of face issues, I wanted to include a link about Synkinesis which showed its effects on patients. Unfortunately, all the sites that I could find that showed patients were those sites of clinics. In that I don't want to give the impression that I am favoring one medical provider over another, I haven't included those links. I would, however, suggest doing an online search. There are a number of clinic sites which describe Synkinesis, suggest therapy, and portray its effects.

And for those of you SSDers who are careless about "good ear" hearing, I wanted to find a link to a site for American Sign Language. What I found was ASL books and ASL schools and classes. Several of the sites depicted the alphabet, but that's the tough way to go. Imagine spelling every word you say.

Finally, did you ever want to declare the world that you are an AN survivor...or congratulate a survivor? Here's a link to AN survivor apparel and gifts.

www.cafepress.com/hellinthehead

NOTES AND OTHER BRAINSTORMS

Made in the USA
San Bernardino, CA
04 December 2019